Messy Connections

This book examines performance practices that involve people in recovery from addiction and offers an understanding of how artistic activity can create social environments – or atmospheres - that support recovery. Focusing on examples of practice from a growing movement of UK-based recovery arts practitioners and performers, it highlights a unique approach to performance that infuses an understanding of lived experiences of addiction and recovery with creative practice. It offers a philosophy of being in recovery that appreciates lived experience, and performance practice, as a dynamic system of interrelations with the human and nonhuman elements that make up the societal settings in which recovery communities struggle to exist. It thereby frames the process of recovery, and recovery-engaged performance, as an affective ecology – a system of messy connections – that enable recovery-friendly environments. Ideas from post-humanist research on addiction, cultural theory on identity and new materialist interpretations of performance practice are applied to highlight the distinct aesthetics, ethics, and politics of this area of performance practice. This study will be of great interest to students and scholars in Applied Theatre, Performance Studies, Critical Arts and Mental Health studies.

Cathy Sloan is Senior Lecturer in Applied and Socially Conscious Theatre at the University of West London.

Routledge Advances in Theatre & Performance Studies

This series is our home for cutting-edge, upper-level scholarly studies and edited collections. Considering theatre and performance alongside topics such as religion, politics, gender, race, ecology, and the avant-garde, titles are characterized by dynamic interventions into established subjects and innovative studies on emerging topics.

The Shakespeare North Playhouse
Replica Theatres and their Uses
Timothy F Keenan

The Art of Entertainment
Popular Performance in Modern British Art, 1880 to 1940
Jason Price

The Routledge Companion to Performance-Related Concepts in Non-European Languages
Erika Fischer-Lichte, Torsten Jost, Astrid Schenka

The Legacy of Stylistic Theatre in the Creation of a Modern Sinhala Drama in Sri Lanka
Lakshmi D Bulathsinghala

Passion and Elegance
How Flamenco and Classical Ballet Met at the Ballets Russes
Barbara Marangon

The Canon in Contemporary Theatre
Plays by Shakespeare, Ibsen, and Brecht in Contemporary Directors' Theatre
Lars Harald Maagerø

Messy Connections
Creating Atmospheres of Addiction Recovery Through Performance Practice
Cathy Sloan

For more information on this series, please visit https://www.routledge.com/Routledge-Research-in-Postcolonial-Literatures/book-series/SE0404

Messy Connections

Creating Atmospheres of Addiction Recovery
Through Performance Practice

Cathy Sloan

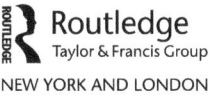

NEW YORK AND LONDON

First published 2024
by Routledge
605 Third Avenue, New York, NY 10158

and by Routledge
4 Park Square, Milton Park, Abingdon, Oxon OX14 4RN

Routledge is an imprint of the Taylor & Francis Group, an informa business

© 2024 Cathy Sloan

The right of Cathy Sloan to be identified as author of this work has been asserted in accordance with sections 77 and 78 of the Copyright, Designs and Patents Act 1988.

All rights reserved. No part of this book may be reprinted or reproduced or utilised in any form or by any electronic, mechanical, or other means, now known or hereafter invented, including photocopying and recording, or in any information storage or retrieval system, without permission in writing from the publishers.

Trademark notice: Product or corporate names may be trademarks or registered trademarks, and are used only for identification and explanation without intent to infringe.

British Library Cataloguing in Publication Data
A catalogue record for this book is available from the British Library

Library of Congress Cataloging-in-Publication Data
A catalog record for this title has been requested

ISBN: 9781032220727 (hbk)
ISBN: 9781032220710 (pbk)
ISBN: 9781003271062 (ebk)

DOI: 10.4324/9781003271062

Typeset in Sabon
by Taylor & Francis Books

For those in recovery, those yet to find recovery and those affected by the addiction of others.

Contents

Acknowledgements   vii

Introduction: Assembling Atmospheres of Recovery through Artistic Practice   1

1   Creating Spaces of Potentiality through Collaborative Theatre-Making   20

2   Facilitating Recovery-Engaged Performance Atmospheres   39

3   Objects of Addiction and Recovery in Artistic Practice   59

4   Place in Recovery-Engaged Performance   77

5   Sustaining Recovery Connections through Creative Kinship   97

6   Coda: Addiction Recovery Arts Network   113

Index   117

Acknowledgements

This book was possible because of the many fruitful and inspirational encounters I've had with fellow artists and practitioners in the field of addiction recovery arts. I wish to acknowledge in particular those who have contributed to the examples and reflections on practice in this book: Liam, Emmer, Charon, Steve, Shiv, Simon Mason, Mark Prest, Matt Steinberg, FK Alexander and Kate McCoy. Posthumous gratitude is extended to Phil Fox and Sonya Hale, both of whom hugely influenced my earlier practice. May their powerful legacies in addiction recovery performance continue to linger. Thanks also to the many other artists-in-recovery and people I have met through the emerging Addiction Recovery Arts network who continue to inspire and fuel my passion for this work.

Many thanks to Zoe Zontou for your guidance and for assisting me with making useful connections as I transitioned from a practitioner to a researcher. I continue to value our ongoing collaborations in developing this area of performance research. Thanks also to Sally Mackey for your warm support and astute mentorship throughout the early development of this research and beyond. Thanks to Selina Busby for your mentorship that led me to this field in the first place. To my doctoral sister, Adelina Ong, thanks for reading drafts and allowing me to test out ideas with a critical friend. To my research degree candidate who follows me into this field, leon clowes, thanks for the insightful conversations that remind me of the importance of sharing this arts practice with others.

Lastly, much gratitude to my family and friends for their support, love and care, especially to my son Ethan, who has brought so much joy and new discovery into my life.

Introduction
Assembling Atmospheres of Recovery through Artistic Practice

Addiction may be regarded as a uniquely human condition. Contemporary societies seem to be riddled with compulsive consumption habits and behaviours, from excessive drinking to social media obsession. Western governments spend significant sums of money on initiatives to address drug abuse, alcoholism and public wellbeing. Private addiction treatment has become a lucrative business. Yet, despite all the research and treatment protocols, addiction continues to cause untimely deaths, damages families and impacts the very environment in which we live. Both Gabor Maté (Maté and Maté 2022, 230) and Marc Lewis (2016, 30) argue from their insights as medical doctors that addiction is a human being's acquired response to some form of adversity, or what we might simply refer to as trauma. While the felt sensations (cravings, highs, withdrawals) and behaviours associated with this response become neurologically ingrained in the way the brain functions and thus become to some extent biological, the cause and, consequently, the cure both feature one key component: social environment.

This book, therefore, is founded on the belief that addiction is an inherent feature of human society and that the everyday realities of this condition are formed by the material surroundings that influence human experience. While the emphasis of much of the discussion in the following chapters leans necessarily on observing human experience, I contend that understanding addiction and the complex process of recovery from it also requires attention to the nonhuman and atmospheric features of our social worlds. Theatrical performance, including a range of arts-based activity, is a unique conduit for attending to the nuance of lived experience and the felt sensations that emerge through interaction with the atmospherics of different social environments. The arts practices discussed in this book highlight the potential of arts-based research to contribute to the review and development of addiction recovery approaches.

As I write this Introduction shortly after the last vestiges of the COVID-19 pandemic, it is all too clear how a nonhuman entity – a virus – can disrupt and take human life on a global scale. During the pandemic, our social worlds were restricted through the implementation of successive lockdowns and social distancing measures. The economic impact of such measures led to significant

DOI: 10.4324/9781003271062-1

loss of income for people working in the service and cultural sectors. Fear, loss and anxiety were but a few of the inevitable sensations experienced during this time, punctuated by moments of heightened awareness of social inequalities such as the Black Lives Matter protests of the summer of 2020. It is unsurprising that a report by the Institute of Alcohol Studies (2022) recorded a significant increase in alcohol consumption and alcohol-related hospital admissions during the period 2020–2021. It is therefore all the more pertinent to consider how environmental conditions impact recovery.

Lockdowns and the social distancing measures enforced to prevent the spread of the virus were likely to exacerbate addiction, leading to increases in relapse or the use of dangerous substitutes for unobtainable substances, and even encouraged the development of new behavioural addictions. For instance, Sujita Kumar Kar et al.'s contribution to the *Elsevier COVID-19 Public Health Emergency Collection* (2020) warned of an increase in the compulsive use of electronic gadgets and media, of relapses caused by interruptions to access of opioid replacement prescriptions, as well as an increase in mental health crises among groups of people affected by addiction who are already vulnerable. In the same series, Felipe Ornell et al. (2020) urged that addiction care must 'be reinforced, not postponed' given the added risk of exposure to COVID-19 among people with substance use dependency. I write, therefore, as we emerge from the collective trauma of a global pandemic, with an appreciation of the urgency of understanding processes of recovery and the practices of survival and resilience that feature in this book. While the discussion focuses specifically on recovery from addiction, insights from these practices of recovery may resonate more broadly as we might reconsider what 'Build Back Better'[1] really means.

Both Anne Wilson Schaef (1987, 5) and Baz Kershaw (cited in Reynolds and Zontou 2014, xi) argued that denial of the systemic factors of addiction prevents recovery by avoiding the source of the problem. Cameron Duff's research on health and society further highlights this point, arguing that attending to the 'assemblage' of addiction (bodies, spaces, affects and relations) leads to a more accurate analysis of how social environment shapes experiences of addiction (2014, 126). Arts activity, through its creative expression of lived experience, can reveal and critique the ways in which society exacerbates addiction and inhibits recovery from it. While I acknowledge that processes of recovery from addiction contain a necessary element of personal development, my discussion of recovery and arts practices in this field deliberately emphasises the sociopolitical context in which they occur. This book challenges the assumption that sustained recovery from addiction is a lone or individual process. Instead, I position addiction and recovery as a collective concern, highlighting the need to move beyond treatment support as entirely focused on individual wellbeing and consider how we operate as a society to more efficiently support collective wellbeing and sustained recovery. Arts practices are an effective way through which to address the social dimension of recovery.

This book offers an approach to performance practice that is recovery-engaged, by which I refer to arts activity that is informed by lived experiences of addiction and is infused by practices of recovery. My discussion draws upon posthumanist research on addiction, cultural theory on identity and new materialist interpretations of performance practice to consider how such contemporary theory might offer additional ways of thinking and doing arts practice with people affected by addiction. By doing so, I not only offer insights into a distinct form of performance practice, but I also highlight the need for such practices to continue to renew, grow and connect. Ultimately, as revealed in the Coda, this book marks the emergence of an Addiction Recovery Arts network through which collaboration, advocacy and mentorship in this unique sector of artistic practice can be facilitated. The examples of performance included throughout this book are drawn from the UK, where my own practice and research is currently based.

Assemblages of Addiction

'Thinking ecologically' (Nicholson 2014, 34) has enabled me to map onto my observations of performance practice an understanding of being in recovery as a living, connected system of survival in the world. It also frames my inquiry into the ways in which recovery-engaged performance practices operate and their potential for growth. Beginning my inquiry with an intention to theorise further the affective experience of this practice, as I had already begun to do (Sloan 2014, 219–230), I developed a deeper understanding of *affect* within the context of process philosophy that shifted my focus from the sensation of affect to attending to systems, or processes, of relation among the human and nonhuman elements involved.

The field of addiction research spans a range of disciplines, including neurology, medical science, psychology, psychiatry, cultural theory, philosophy and performance studies.[2] While acknowledging the important contribution of each discipline in our attempts to understand addiction, for the purpose of my discussion of arts practice in this book the *posthumanist* or *new materialist* approaches to addiction research are useful in how they highlight the environmental contexts in which lived experience occurs (Duff 2014; Dennis and Farrugia 2017). These environmental elements include nonhuman features, such as place, objects, social structures and economics, as well as other humans. The way in which a person interacts with these elements can be considered, according to affect theory, as affective relations; sensorial and energetic exchanges that influence a person's response and sense of who they are in the world. Performance practice, like addiction, is a sensorial experience and is, therefore, a productive mechanism for examining the environmental players in scenes (or assemblages) of addiction and for creating new, recovery-orientated social atmospheres.

In their editorial for *Drugged Pleasures*, Fay Dennis and Adrian Farrugia highlighted how new materialist readings of drug use illustrate the need for a revision of current drug policy to adopt an ethics of care in which the contexualised experience of the drug consumer matters (2017, 88). The radical shift they offer, in my view, is a reorientating of addiction research and policy to the vantage point of the body affected by addiction, and its interactions with objects, substances and its surroundings, rather than imposing decisions made from an external diagnosis on an essentialised 'addict' body that inevitably limits agency and marginalises.

To elaborate on how this is achieved, it is useful to embrace Duff's concept of health as an assemblage. Duff uses Gilles Deleuze's concept of assemblage, specifically the ideas of immanence and 'becoming'. He applies these concepts to the experience of addiction to challenge neoliberal concepts of health that rely on essentialising judgements based on biological criteria and classifications of social and structural phenomena (Duff 2014, 5). For Deleuze and Felix Guattari, the concept of immanence was the appreciation of the emergence of 'immediate, perpetual, instantaneous exchange' between thought and body (1994, 38). Brian Massumi developed this concept further and argued that *becoming* is pre-cognitive in that during the time-lapse between 'intensity' (a felt sensation) and consciousness what happens is too quick to have registered as actually happening and is thus virtual (2002, 30).

Duff applied the concepts of immanence and becoming, citing both Deleuze and Massumi's interpretations, to reframe concepts of health and wellness to acknowledge that the body 'emerges in a multiplicity of dynamic singularities (affects, events and relations)' that later settle in the familiar form that we recognise (2014, 13).

In the context of addressing approaches to health in relation to addiction, Duff critiqued predominant approaches in addiction research and treatment that proliferate 'causal' explanations of drug misuse that 'inform and endorse the vast apparatus' used to solve the problem (2014, 125). Proposing a shift in analysis towards addressing the connections of the body within an assemblage of space, place, bodies, affects and relations (127), he offered a flexible framework with which to consider not only the nuanced ways in which social, economic and political factors contribute to addiction, but also allows for individual variation in the way in which bodies are affected by, and respond in relation to, the assemblage differently. The concept of addiction as an assemblage is particularly useful for the discussions of performance in this book in appreciating how a theatrical event is composed, as well as enabling a more adequate account of subjective differences in the manner that bodies are also gendered, racialised, or additionally 'othered' in accordance with established notions of a generalised 'norm'.

Duff identifies three layers of the assemblage framework that, in my view, correspond well with performance practice. These are (i) spatial relations; (ii) modes of embodiment; and (iii) affective atmospheres (Duff 2014, 132). His identification of a need for more nuanced accounts of the 'real' experience of drug use (143) highlights the transdisciplinary gap within which this book sits in demonstrating how arts practice can assemble and present the relational patterns of lived experience of addiction. I also consider his point to be reinforced by attempts by other researchers who, following Duff, have endeavoured to reassemble the material experience of addiction.

For instance, Dennis used Deleuze's concept of becoming to challenge the presumption that the consumption of heroin by a person in active addiction is abnormal. Rather, she shared the narrative of 'Mya', a heroin user, to reveal how her lived experience of taking heroin is, in contrast, an effort towards 'becoming normal' (Dennis 2016). Dennis argued that Mya's narrative challenges ideas of recovery purported by current health and public policy that assume that people remove themselves from drugs in order to regain their 'normal' self. It is evident in Mya's narrative that heroin forms part of the process by which her body forms its relation with the world around her. It constitutes part of her sense of who she is and how she functions. Dennis, with Farrugia, developed this understanding of the contingent experience of drug consumption to argue for a shift in ethical and political imperatives to research, practice and policy away from 'stagnant morals' towards a more caring responsibility for how realities, and marginalisation, are produced (2017, 88). They proposed that openness to learning from the lived experience of drug users requires us to 'expand our concerns beyond reducing harm towards living well' (91). I interpret from this that they also invite a re-evaluation of what is considered to be living well by not only accounting for the differing experiences of other bodies but also accepting that such bodies and their relational assemblages should be valued as much as any other. Throughout the following chapters of this book, I elaborate upon concepts of 'living well' in relation to arts practice.

Beyond Disease and Criminalisation

Yet much drug and addiction policy at government level still relies on the traditional medical model of addiction as a disease and strategies involving the criminal justice system. Current policy on addiction treatment that influences the provision of funding for addiction treatment services still draws heavily on the concept of addiction as a disease. Alan Leshner's influential publication, written while he was director of the US National Institute for Drug Abuse (NIDA) from 1994–2001, defined addiction as a 'chronic, relapsing [brain] disease' (1997, 45). While I agree with Lewis's criticism of the disease model as a limited interpretation of the nuanced discoveries made by neurological scientists, I am nonetheless wary of rejecting the disease model (or the medical model) entirely given that this approach to addiction has led to increased support and funding for addiction treatment and challenges the criminalisation of people affected by addiction. For instance, the UK's most recent drug strategy refers to addiction as a 'chronic health condition' that requires long-term support and commits to increased investment in services that will provide mental and physical healthcare, housing and employment as well as substance abuse treatment (HM Government 2021, 31).[3] Similarly,

NIDA's 2021–2025 strategic plan positions recovery treatment within the context of public health.

Beyond the science of addiction research, it is useful to note that the adoption of the concept of addiction as a disease has been used productively by the Twelve Steps of Alcoholics Anonymous (and AA's other associate organisations such as Narcotics Anonymous or Cocaine Anonymous). The exact degree to which AA's founding members intended to support the notion that is the current medicalised 'disease model' is unclear and, in fact, is disputed.[4] Nevertheless, Steps 1 and 2 do imply acceptance from those following the programme that they are suffering from some form of malady over which they have no control. Philosopher Gabriel Segal offered a more recent analysis of the Twelve Steps to demonstrate how the programme supports recovery from 'disease', making comparative links to neurological research (2017, 379–380).

Yet Hall et al. have argued that there is an overemphasis on the brain disease model that has failed either to lead to a 'cure' or to adequately cater to the complex interaction of factors impacting neurobiology that suggest that evidence from other disciplines, such as social science, should not be obscured by an overemphasis on biomedical science (2015, 108). I contend that research by practitioners in recovery-engaged performance can also add useful insights into the contextualised, lived experiences of addiction and recovery.

Treatment policies have developed in recent years and it appears that it is widely accepted, in the UK and the US, that treatment programmes should treat a person holistically, providing therapies and counselling that might address psychological wellbeing as well as support from social service agencies, such as housing, to assist with reintegration back into 'society'. Nonetheless, continued social stigma and inadequately funded public treatment services mean that addiction support is often inaccessible to those in most need. For instance, in *Gendering Addiction*, Nancy Campbell and Elizabeth Ettorre highlighted that women, as well as people from ethnic minorities and other marginalised groups, including the LGBTQ+ community and those with disabilities, were unable to access effective support (2014, 1). They attributed this to generic approaches based upon a generalised norm that particularly suited white, hetero males, and consequently argued for the creation of new approaches that acknowledged the multidimensional narratives of lived experiences that are outside of the generic norm (1). It is important, in my discussions of recovery-engaged performance practice, to highlight the systemic value systems that reinforce prejudices and cause further exclusion, thereby inhibiting access to addiction support and inhibiting recovery.

Western culture also continues to stigmatise people affected by addiction to illicit substances as immoral in that criminalisation remains a key aspect of drug strategy. For instance, Hall et al. noted that the even NIDA's brain disease approach has had insufficient impact on US drug policy that is still overinvested in law enforcement efforts to decrease drug supply (2015, 108). Coincidentally, while the UK's current drug strategy commits to meeting the needs of those who 'have not had an effective [treatment] service in the past, including ethnic minority backgrounds and women', much of the overall strategy emphasises a criminal justice approach (HM Government 2021).

The prohibitionist policy of the War on Drugs and its consequent criminalisation of people addicted to what are deemed to be illicit substances reflects a governmental approach that ascribes deviancy to those not considered to conform to notions of good citizenship. This, in turn, impacts the social context and psychosocial experience of people affected by addiction. Officially launched in a speech delivered by US President Nixon in June 1971, the War on Drugs materialised as the US policy on drug control that was subsequently endorsed worldwide, influencing policy towards the prohibition and control of the drug trade internationally. Those addicted to prohibited substances are criminalised and controlled via the judicial system of their respective countries. In fact, through the laws of prohibition, they are not just positioned as morally deviant, but are caught in a cycle in which they will inevitably continue to contravene the law in order to both procure and use the substance on which they have a dependency.

A report facilitated by UK drugs reform charity Release, entitled *A Quiet Revolution*, highlighted that, despite an annual expenditure of approximately £100 billion on law enforcement approaches to drug policy, there has been a continued increase in drug use, prison populations and drug-related deaths (Eastwood et al. 2016, 6). It emphasised the disproportionate impact of criminalisation upon ethnic minorities within the UK (6). Indeed, its subsequent report, *The Colour of Injustice*, drew on statistics gathered during the Lammy Review[5] of the UK criminal justice system to prove that 'stop and search' police strategies are applied predominantly to black and Asian groups (Shiner et al. 2018, vi) For instance, according to statistics from 2016/2017, black people were five times more likely to be searched than white people pro rata (vi). Yet policing reports reveal that the 'find' rate for drugs was lower for black people than for white people, indicating an unjustified bias in search targets (vi). The report also noted racial disparity in rates of prosecution and custodial sentencing, stating that drug policing was a 'key driver' of ethnic disparities throughout the criminal justice system (viii and 61).

Nonetheless, as *A Quiet Revolution* has revealed, there is a growing shift towards policy reform that favours decriminalisation as a more effective approach (Eastwood et al. 2016, 6). Both the Global Commission on Drug Policy and the United Nations Office on Drugs and Crime have advocated decriminalisation, although the UN quickly rescinded its 2015 publication declaring its support for reform (7). While it would seem that there is growing pressure to adopt policy reform, particularly from countries most affected by aggressive prohibition measures such as Guatemala, Columbia and Mexico, decriminalisation has been met with resistance in the west, particularly in the UK (7). Yet prohibitionist policy neither elevates nor prevents the psychosocial factors that influence addiction. Rather, it creates barriers to care in how it stigmatises some bodies as criminal and, more poignantly, in how the inequitable application of the justice system reinforces institutionalised prejudices along lines of race and class.

The posthumanist and new materialist approaches to addiction research, discussed earlier, are therefore crucial to reviewing policies, practices and services by shifting priorities of what or, indeed, who 'matters'. Through approaching addiction as an assemblage, we can appreciate more fully how systemic features of society, including systems of law and order, can exacerbate the psychosocial factors of addiction. Indeed, through the sensorial experience of arts activity, we can create new recovery-orientated assemblages that are more fluid in how they can respond to the nuances of lived experience.

Towards Atmospheres of Recovery

As Dennis and Farrugia have argued, by de-centring moralistic notions of harm, it is possible to imagine 'possibilities for new and more caring subjectivities, bodies, substances and concepts' (2017, 91). They argue for more 'situated' interventions based on the understanding of how any addiction-based activity is situated within, and emerges from, an assemblage of bodies, objects and space-times (91) Such interventions might include the provision of monitored drug consumption rooms.[6] For Duff, recovery is best supported by altering the context of the 'assemblage of addiction'; a combination of spatial relations, modes of embodiment and affective atmospheres (2014, 132). The spatial relations to which he referred denoted the manner in which the surrounding context of place, time, socio-economic and environmental features 'fold' into the event of substance use or addiction-based behaviour (135). He recognised the changeable nature of these contexts as also created by the bodies in them. With particular relevance to this book, these concepts informed Duff's understanding of the experience of recovery as a process of 'becoming well' through an emerging capacity to manipulate one's interactions with the surrounding environment (2016, 58).

The word 'recovery' is, in my view, a misnomer, with its implications of a return to or a recovering of some normative notion of static wellbeing. My own approach to the concept of recovery and, subsequently, recovery-engaged performance practice appreciates the existential crisis that is instigated by the 'rock bottom' of addiction[7] and, thereby, the affective dimension of being-in-recovery. This process of 'becoming well' is not only navigation of creating new, less harmful forms of interaction with the surrounding environment, but also involves the development of an embodied understanding of one's own sense of *being* in the world. Narratives of addiction recovery shared by the people I have met through my theatre practice over the years entail a combination of processes of change involving the personal (mind and body), the environment (social and geographical) and the spiritual (relationship with a higher power). Engagement in these acts of change are largely an ongoing effort towards finding balance in how one is affected by or affects the world around them. Given this existential aspect of addiction recovery, it follows that my discussion of recovery-engaged arts practice attends to the ways in which creative activity can enable expressions of the affective, sensorial dimension of *being-in-recovery*.

I appreciate the lived experience of addiction as involving a loop of extreme sensations, behavioural and thinking processes, in which a person may find themselves caught within an entropic cycle. The perpetual loop of thinking and behaviour manifested in the 'graft-score-use' process of active addiction renders a person unable to cease activity that is increasingly detrimental to their capacity to engage in the world around them and is ultimately a threat to their health and wellbeing.[8] Recovery, therefore, entails practices that foster a balance in how interactions (affective relations) with the surrounding environment are experienced in a way that increases a body's capacity to affect and be affected by avoiding the swing towards extremes that disrupt and divert 'becoming well'. This involves the development of new approaches to relation with the world around us that are also resilient to the inevitable painful sensations of life and its associated losses. It includes a process of active and embodied learning of strategies for survival founded upon intra- and interpersonal discoveries of less harmful ways to respond to felt sensations. Yet given the relational dimension of any process of being in the world, it is pertinent to consider how the surrounding environments may increase or decrease a body's capacity for recovery. The chapters that follow reveal how arts practice can both reveal the ways in which society inhibits recovery and also supports participants to explore and strengthen their own recovery-orientated experiences.

The felt experience of identity is also a recurring theme in recovery circles; specifically, a transition from 'addict' to 'recovery' identity. The lived experience of recovery entails an existential dimension of developing a sense of self following active addiction. Sometimes this might be viewed as a form of rebirth, marked by the celebration of sobriety birthdays or sober anniversaries. It is important, therefore, to understand how affect relates to the lived experience of identity. The relational construction of identity was much discussed in the 1990s by key cultural theorists working in the fields of critical race and gender studies, such as Stuart Hall (1997) and Judith Butler (1990). For my interpretation of the affective experience of being-in-recovery, Erin Manning's interpretation of affect as a force that lures relation enables an understanding of how affect contributes to the lived perception of human experiences of identity. She proposed that identity is 'the pinnacle of a relational field tuning in to a certain constellation' (2013, 17). In other words, the body tunes into its surroundings through sensory interaction. The event of human perception is a momentary awareness of the positionality of one's body in relation to its surroundings, which may seem static.

This concept of the felt sensation of identity encapsulates the paradox of lived experience. Our quotidian routines often involve strong attachments to certain identities, a sense of self that may seem static. Yet experiences of identity shift according to changes in social or geographical context. For instance, migration to a different country shifts one's experience of identity in relation to the cultural practices and values of the new social context. Additionally, as we encounter difference or learn from new experience, our perception of ourselves and the world around us changes. Manning's discussion of identity encourages an appreciation of the paradox of identity through which we register a sense of self that remains the same, while simultaneously recognising that this is contingent and subject to change as we grow and develop. This appreciation of fluidity in identity offers hope to those in addiction recovery and arts practice is an effective mechanism for exploring a shifting sense of self.

Sara Ahmed's affective economy reminds us of the role of emotion in how humans experience affect and identity. For Ahmed, emotion is how we come into contact with objects and other bodies in the world (2014, 8). The somatic sensation of emotion orientates a body towards or away from others and therefore moves beyond the personal to represent an aspect of relational, social experience. Emotion is a crucial orientating force for humans in how it generates a perceptual viewpoint and, consequently, a sense of identity. For people in recovery, emotion is a valence of feeling that they must navigate during their process of recovery. A phrase often used by participants in my own theatre-making sessions is that after getting clean, 'I had to learn how to feel my feelings'. This initial phase of recovery often entails learning how to manage the experience of unpleasant feelings that can often seem overwhelming and may even trigger relapse (Burgess 2017, 313; Segal 2017, 379–380).

Lingering affect, such as transgenerational trauma, can also contribute to social environments that inhibit recovery and may even fuel addiction. Nicolas Abraham and Maria Torok's study of 'transgenerational haunting' highlights the role of affect in how the effects of trauma are transferred from one generation to the next (cited in Clough and Halley 2007, 9). They argue that trauma itself has no conscious memory and so becomes an embodied memory (9). Such work advocates for a better understanding of how the lingering affects of lived experience can impact a person, indeed a whole family or community, across an extended time frame. This resonates with Maté's contention in *The Realm of Hungry Ghosts* that causes of addiction have historic roots (2013, 17). Marsh et al.'s (2021) study of addiction treatment approaches with Indigenous Canadians in Ontario also highlights the connection between transgenerational trauma, including the legacies of harm endured under colonisation, and substance abuse. It is critical, therefore, that my analysis of the affective capacity of theatrical performance and arts activity comprehends the sociopolitical and cultural influences on affect.

Duff proposed that opportunities for 'becoming well' might be better facilitated through the 'staging of atmospheres of recovery' that understand the way in which recovery is supported through an 'attunement' to the way in which affects, spaces and bodies operate to enhance or inhibit individual experiences (2016, 58). Rather than focusing on the championing of personal recovery targets that are grounded 'too much in subjective labour', he argued that emphasis should be placed on cultivating spaces that offer atmospheres of recovery (62). Such atmospheres enable the ebb and flow of sociality, hope, belonging and other positive pro-social sensations (67–69).

Across the UK, there are recovery services that provide social activities for people in recovery from addiction. For instance, there are a variety of local recovery cafés that are often attached to addiction services or charities, such as Blenheim Community Drug Project's Shine café in Haringey, London, or Cascade Creative Recovery's café in Brighton. Organisations such as Build on Belief and The Firm[9] facilitate weekend social activities, including arts and sports activities, at treatment centres across London. There is even a 'dry' bar, The Brink, managed by Action on Addiction in Liverpool. Nonetheless, such provision is limited to local initiatives or specific aftercare treatment programmes so that access is not equitably available to people in recovery nationally. This is particularly evident in the lack of provision of recovery activities for people who might benefit from social activities tailored for specific identity groups. For example, Club Soda facilitate 'Queers without Beers' evenings in London and Manchester to provide an outlet for members of the LGBTQ+ community to socialise within an alcohol-free social space. There are also recovery musical groups, such as the Rising Voices choir in Bristol and the New Note Orchestra in Brighton.

While it is evident that many treatment services facilitate social activities as part of their programmes, there is a need for the wider availability of potential recovery support networks beyond the scope of initial treatment programmes. Given that addiction research accepts that recovery is a perpetual process, it should follow that access to atmospheres of recovery needs to exist within and across the intersections of local communities. Duff also highlighted the importance of enduring atmospheres that can be sustained in everyday practices and encounters (72). It is insufficient, therefore, to evaluate recovery services on the basis of individualised achievements of recovery targets, such as sobriety, rehousing or re-entering employment. Instead, recovery approaches must consider public health as a collective concern in how the patterns and structures of society formulate atmospheres in which all bodies can live well.

Currently, within the UK, there are organisations that highlight the need for collective change. For instance, Faces and Voices of Recovery (FAVOR) UK and the Scottish Recovery Consortium advocate for recognition of a recovery community. Through organising annual 'recovery walks', lobbying local government and disseminating information on issues related to addiction and recovery, I consider that both show the potential to cultivate atmospheres of recovery in the public domain. By resisting marginalisation through increasing the visibility and representation of the perspectives and expertise of people who have survived addiction, they demonstrate how recovery communities can cohabitate with, and even benefit, mainstream society. Moreover, the emergent field of recovery arts, particularly the launch of the Recoverist Manifesto in 2015 (Parkinson 2015), has utilised performance to publicly manifest variations of recovery community, a community that acknowledges its diverse intersections of identity and experience.

An Ecology of 'Life-Living'

'Becoming well' involves affective attunements with others and oneself to generate new modes of being that acknowledge dissonance and difference in order to develop less extreme strategies for living. Manning's concept of 'life-living' extends these ideas to a politics of interdependency and collaboration. Her philosophy for life-living refuses to 'privilege this life over that', while also honouring 'the singular event we call our life' (2016, 8). Consequently, the ecology of practice I offer in the following chapters considers how relations of care are nurtured through arts practices to acknowledge our collective interdependency on others, human and nonhuman, to promote systems, or communities, which enable capacities for recovery.

Performance practice, specifically with people in recovery from addiction, might be considered as an affective ecology that can generate an atmosphere of recovery. Attending to modes of relation during the creation and staging of performances can generate an affective ecology that is recovery-engaged. Being-in-recovery is an ecological process, an effort towards equilibrium in response to the inevitable antagonisms of the surrounding world to enable continued evolution towards less harmful forms of thinking, feeling and doing. Translating this ecology into an observation of systems of *messy connection*, it becomes possible to identify the features of theatrical performance and arts practice that address both the felt sensation of participation and the yet to be discovered potential of creative explorations of being-in-recovery.

Messy Connections

Theatre and performance practice is especially primed to instigate and perpetuate connection with people, spaces and things. In my attention to arts practices in this book, I observe the ways in which connection – or affective interaction – occurs. This is relevant in that the development of positive, less harmful connections to people, oneself, objects, space and place is a key aspect of the journey towards recovery from addiction. As journalist Johann Hari claimed, 'the opposite of addiction is connection' (2015). Often, during the active cycle of addiction, there is an experience of disconnection with others as the compulsive relationship with the object of addiction takes precedence. Moving beyond social isolation is, therefore, a crucial component of 'becoming well.'

The correlation of connections with addiction and recovery is, nonetheless, not a novel concept and is iterated by other writers who account for the first-hand experience of addiction and recovery. For instance, Gabor Maté emphasised the negative impact of the absence of a healthy connection with a primary caregiver in childhood (2013, 154–156). Drawing on Panksepp et al.'s neurological research, he argued that the inhibition of developing strong attachments to a parent figure as an infant led to neurochemical, and subsequently behavioural, change that accumulated into a tendency in adulthood to seek alternative sources of soothing connection (154–156). To substantiate this claim, Maté's *In the Realm of Hungry Ghosts: Close Encounters with Addiction* (2013) provided several narratives from patients he had treated as a medical doctor to illustrate how their desire for soothing connection had materialised into addiction to substances and, often, abusive relationships with others.

This has also been observed in more popular contexts. The celebrity Russell Brand has particularly emphasised the role of connection in his own writing on recovery (2017). Addiction, he argued, is an attempt to 'solve the problem of disconnection, alienation, tepid despair' (14). Segal elaborated on the Twelve Steps of recovery as a process through which self-absorption and egocentric perspectives are altered to develop 'a psychologically healthy involvement with the world around you and the other sentient, feeling beings that inhabit it' (2014, 1 and 17). Modes of connection are also a prominent feature of other forms of recovery programme, as demonstrated by Leighton's research on the counselling and peer group processes of the SMART recovery model 10 (2017, 177).

Adopting Duff's assemblage approach to addiction, I frame the performance practices discussed in this book as an affective ecology to denote the ways in which performance activity instigates relation with other bodies, objects and space, through a sensorial or energetic experience. Theatrical performance and arts-based activity are very much considered to be affective experiences. Since the turn of the 21st century, scholarship in theatre and performance has increasingly applied concepts from affect theory to examine the sensorial dimension of performance spectatorship (Dolan 2005), participation (Thompson 2011), atmospherics (Alston and Welton 2019) and politics (Fragkou 2019). My discussion of affect – or the affective interrelations – of theatrical performance and arts practice in this book, however, purposefully shifts away from an emphasis on affect theory and instead, as Manning has done, envelops an appreciation of affect within process philosophy (2013). Affect, therefore, becomes a contextualised aspect of understanding the felt experience of the process of *being* and the relational influences of identity, which are crucial to a nuanced understanding of the varied experiences of addiction and recovery across different sociocultural settings.

Throughout this book, I therefore set out a framework for analysing recovery-engaged arts as an affective ecology; systems of practice that simultaneously facilitate and reveal physicalised encounters with other people, space, objects, place and sociopolitical atmospheres. I emphasise the affective dimension of being-in-recovery which underpins my premise that arts activity is an effective mechanism for not only generating 'atmospheres of recovery', but also supporting continued connections to recovery community post-treatment which in turn promotes sustained practices of recovery. In particular, I address examples of recovery-engaged performance activity to illustrate the ways in which connection operates through affective and emotive encounters. Duff's concept of 'atmospheres of recovery' invites further exploration of how recovery communities and identities might emerge through collaborative artistic expression. Rather than impose a neoliberal agenda for recovery that inevitably caters for a generalised norm, arts practices that are attuned to the affective experiences of people in recovery can support a deeper understanding of the varied processes of 'becoming well' (Duff 2016, 58).

As recovery is an ongoing process of becoming well, it is useful to frame the existential state of being-in-recovery as a 'body-in-process' in the manner that Manning describes the body as a 'relational field' that experiences attunement or antagonism with its surroundings (2013, 19). Being-in-recovery is, therefore, a perpetual, relational practice, navigating the affective dimensions of one's experience of the world to develop a way of being that incorporates practices that support a recovery-orientated existence. This philosophical approach to the experience of recovery informs my discussion of a recovery-engaged orientation to performance practice.

To translate my philosophical framing of being-in-recovery and, subsequently, recovery-engaged performance practice as an affective ecology more closely to everyday experience, I use the phrase *messy connections*. I prefix connections with *messy* to denote the bodily sensations involved that are simultaneously difficult to record and are emotive, volatile and potentially antagonistic. *Messy Connections* is used, therefore, as a metaphorical device that equates to the experiential processes of creative performance activity as well as the nonlinear, emotive and conflictual progress of recovery from addiction. The reference to messy connections in this book combines Ahmed's discussion of visceral and emotional bodily experience (2014, 210) with Manning's concept of mess as the 'unquantifiable' aspect of the 'not-quite-yet' emerged (2016, 29). My discussion of the examples presented in this book not only appreciates the felt sensations that occur in the creating, performing and spectating, but also considers the potential future developments that are not yet known. My purpose is not to quantify this practice, but to reveal insights and observations which might encourage new or further developments in addiction recovery arts practice.

I attempt, in the chapters that follow, to capture a snapshot of the 'messy connections' of the field of recovery-engaged practices in the UK. These connections are messy in their simultaneous constellation of personal experiences of recovery from addiction, modes of belonging to communities of recovery and ranges of arts practices amid wider sociopolitical attachments to the criminalisation or medicalisation of many people affected by addiction. It seems apt to also share my own connection to this field of performance practice. My practice in recovery arts began as a practitioner with Outside Edge Theatre Company in London. Outside Edge was, at the time, the only theatre company in the UK focused exclusively on creating theatre with and by people in recovery from addiction for public audiences. I worked closely with the founder of the company, Phil Fox, who drew upon his own recovery from heroin addiction in his practice as a writer and director. During my time with the company, I created and facilitated a broad range of theatre projects addressing issues related to addiction which were based in contexts such as drug and alcohol treatment, education, mental health and prison settings. I was also involved in the creation and production of the company's public performance work, some of which was performed in professional theatre spaces. Simultaneously, I embarked on my own recovery journey. After Fox's death from a heart attack in June 2014, I stepped into his role as Artistic Director. With the support of my colleagues and the board of trustees, I guided the company through the immediate crisis that was precipitated by the sudden loss of Fox. In 2015, I resigned from the company in order to pursue doctoral research. Since completing my doctoral study, I have co-founded the Addiction Recovery Arts network, the *Performing Recovery* magazine and curated a number of recovery arts events.

I provide this information about my career in order to reveal my attachments to the field of practice discussed in this book. This has provided me with access to performers and practitioners who know me, or know of me, or know the lineage of practice (with Phil Fox) that my experience is connected to. It is important for me to acknowledge, therefore, the simultaneous roles I have navigated in the conduct of this research as practitioner, researcher, colleague and peer. I am very aware of my obligation to, and attachments with, the practices in this book. I do not, however, interpret this as a sense of duty through which I am bound to exert some sort of control or judgement over practice. Rather, I recognise the ways in which I am able to do this research in the way that I do because of the attachments I have to it.

Each chapter of this book attends to particular modes of relation that reveal a recovery-engaged ethico-political orientation to performance practice. I highlight forms of interaction with others, space, objects, place, social and temporal atmospheres made possible by theatrical and creative arts activity to offer you, the reader, some insight into the unique perspectives on the lived experience of recovery from addiction revealed through these activities. Ultimately, I propose that arts activity, by evoking 'atmospheres of recovery', can instigate, support and sustain communities of recovery.

Notes

1 'Build Back Better: Our Plan for Growth' (March 2021) was a policy paper produced by the incumbent UK Conservative government outlining plans to support the country's economic recovery post-pandemic. I use it here to highlight the multiple and polysemic references to the term 'recovery' during the pandemic.
2 Paul Blobaum's review of the literature on addiction treatment in medical sciences and psychiatry journals noted a total of 40,957 articles, demonstrating the large extent of research on addiction in these disciplines (2013, 109). This book is less concerned with the medical treatment of addiction and so does not attempt a survey of this literature.

16 *Introduction*

3 This policy paper by the incumbent UK government (*From Harm to Hope: A Ten-Year Drugs Plan to Cut Crime and Save Lives*) also reveals a re-emphasis on criminal justice approaches to restricting access to illicit drugs. It adopts an approach that drug abuse is a 'problem for all society and that all government must deal with it', while drawing a clear division between respectable members of society and 'offenders' who require punishment for their crimes (HM Government 2021, 3).

4 Ernest Kurtz disputed the assumptions attributed to AA that presume that the Twelve Steps are based on the premise of addiction as a disease, in particular the concept of an allergy that is spoken of in AA circles (2002, 5).

5 The Lammy Review, chaired by David Lammy (elected Member of Parliament for Tottenham 2000–), was an independent review of the treatment of black and minority ethnic people within the UK criminal justice system. The report was published and made available on the UK government website in September 2017.

6 Drug consumption rooms are facilities where illicit drugs can be used under the supervision of trained staff. These have been operating in some European countries since 1986. The Advisory Council on the Misuse of Drugs published a report in December 2016 recommending medically supervised drug consumption clinics as a potentially effective strategy, among other opioid reduction methods, to reduce the growing rate of drug misuse deaths (Advisory Council on the Misuse of Drugs 2016). In England drug deaths involving opioids rose by 58% from 2012–2016. The official response from the UK government, at that time, dismissed the proposal. Although the Scottish Parliament voted in favour of opening a 'fix room' in Glasgow, plans were stalled by refusal from the UK Home Office to make the necessary changes in legislation to allow it to function. The UK Faculty of Public Health renewed demand for the piloting of drug consumptions rooms in an open letter to the British government in December 2021 in respond to the publication of the government's new drug strategy. A pilot scheme was eventually given clearance to operate in 2023.

7 The term 'rock bottom' is used as a reference to the phrase commonly used by people in recovery as the point of extreme crisis in active addiction that instigates the decision to seek addiction treatment. This tends to represent a turning point during active addiction that can be precipitated by a financial, psychological, health or judicial crisis. I suggest, however, that the lived experience of a rock bottom is simultaneously an existential crisis in that it is associated with questioning what it means to exist in this world and questions identity. For some, there may be several experiences of a rock bottom before recovery is sustained.

8 The phrase 'graft-score-use' is a common idiom of active addiction which refers to the repetitive cycle of activity involved. The word 'graft' denotes the means by which someone might acquire the money to purchase their addictive substance of choice. 'Score' refers to the purchase of this substance and 'use' indicates the action of taking the substance. It is possible to apply this cycle to all forms of addiction, substituting 'substance' for whichever object is the focus of activity.

9 The Firm was based at the same premises as Outside Edge, on Munster Road, London, until lack of sufficient funding forced the organisation to stop functioning. Nevertheless, those involved continue to provide a similar service as part of the Barons Court Project within the same borough of London. This indicates how difficult it is for small, local projects to function in the long term.

10 SMART (Self Management and Recovery Training) is a community-based programme that provides training and strategies for people to address addiction issues. This includes cognitive behaviour therapy approaches as well as other motivational tools to support change in lifestyle.

References

Advisory Council on the Misuse of Drugs (2016) Reducing opioid- related deaths in the UK. Available at: chromeextension://efaidnbmnnnibpcajpcglclefindmkaj/https://kar.kent.ac.uk/62867/1/ACMD-Drug-Related-Deaths-Report-161212.pdf.

Ahmed, S. (2014) *The cultural politics of emotion*. 2nd ed. Edinburgh: Edinburgh University Press.

Alston, A. and Welton, M. (2019) *Theatre in the dark: Shadow, gloom and blackout in contemporary theatre*. London and New York: Methuen Drama.

Barton, N., Leighton, T., Gregory, K., Anderson, D. and Tomson, A. (2015) 'Research strategy 2015'. Action on Addiction. Available at: www.actiononaddiction.org.uk (accessed 19 October 2017).

Bennett, J. (2010) *Vibrant matter: A political ecology of things*. Durham, NC: Duke University Press.

Blobaum, P.M. (2013) 'Mapping the literature of addictions treatment', *Journal of the Medical Library Association*, 101 (2), pp. 101–109. Available at: https://doi.org/10.3163/1536-5050.101.2.005.

Brand, R. (2017) *Recovery: Freedom from your addictions*. London: Bluebird.

Burgess, B. (2017) 'The blindfold of addiction', in N. Heather and G. Segal (eds), *Addiction and choice: Rethinking the relationship*. Oxford and New York: Oxford University Press, pp. 307–324.

Butler, J. (2006) *Gender trouble: feminism and the subversion of identity*. New York: Routledge.

Campbell, N. and Ettorre, E. (2014) *Gendering addiction*. Basingstoke and New York: Palgrave Macmillan.

Clough, P.T. and Halley, J.O. (eds) (2007) *The affective turn: Theorizing the social*. Durham, NC: Duke University Press.

Deleuze, G. and Guattari, F. (1994) *What is philosophy?* New York: Columbia University Press.

Dennis, F. and Farrugia, A. (2017) 'Materialising drugged pleasures: Practice, politics, care', *International Journal of Drug Policy*, 49, pp. 86–91.

Dolan, J. (2005) *Utopia in performance: Finding hope at the theater*. Ann Arbor: University of Michigan Press.

Duff, C. (2014) *Assemblages of health: Deleuze's empiricism and the ethology of life*. New York: Springer.

Duff, C. (2016) 'Atmospheres of recovery: Assemblages of health', *Environment and Planning A*, 48 (1), pp. 58–74. Available at: https://doi.org/10.1177/0308518X15603222.

Eastwood, N., Fox, E. and Rosmarin, A. (2016) *A quiet revolution: Drug decriminalisation across the globe*. London: Release.

Ettorre, E. (2015) 'Embodied deviance, gender, and epistemologies of ignorance: Re-visioning drugs use in a neurochemical, unjust world', *Substance Use & Misuse*, 50 (6), pp. 794–805. Available at: https://doi.org/10.3109/10826084.2015.978649.

Fragkou, M. (2019) *Ecologies of precarity in twenty-first century theatre: Politics, affect, responsibility*. London: Methuen Drama.

Hall, S. (ed.) (1997) *Representation: Cultural representations and signifying practices*. London and Thousand Oaks, CA: SAGE in association with the Open University.

Hall, W., Carter, A. and Forlini, C. (2015) 'The brain disease model of addiction: Is it supported by the evidence and has it delivered on its promises?', *The Lancet*

Psychiatry, 2 (1), pp. 105–110. Available at: https://doi.org/10.1016/S2215-0366(14)00126-6.

Hari, J. (2015) 'Everything you think you know about addiction is wrong'. TED Talk, London, June. Available at: https://www.ted.com/talks/johann_hari_every thing_you_think_you_know_about_addiction_is_wrong?language=en (accessed 19 July 2017).

HM Government (2021) *From harm to hope: A 10-year drugs plan to cut crime and save lives*. London: HMSO. Available at: https://www.gov.uk/government/publica tions/from-harm-to-hope-a-10-year-drugs-plan-to-cut-crime-and-save-lives (accessed 2 September 2022).

Institute of Alcohol Studies (2022) *The COVID hangover: Addressing long-term health impacts of changes in alcohol consumption during the pandemic*, July. Available at: chrome-extension://efaidnbmnnnibpcajpcglclefindmkaj/https://www.ias.org.uk/wp-con tent/uploads/2022/07/The-COVID-Hangover-report-July-2022.pdf.

Kar, S.K., Arafat, S.M.Y., Sharma, P., Dixit, A., Marthoenis, M. and Kabir, R. (2020) 'COVID-19 pandemic and addiction: Current problems and future concerns', *Asian Journal of Psychiatry*, 51, p. 102064. Available at: https://doi.org/10.1016/j.ajp.2020.102064.

Kershaw, B. (2007) *Theatre ecology: Environments and performance events*. Cambridge and New York: Cambridge University Press.

Kurtz, E. (2002) 'Alcoholics Anonymous and the disease concept of alcoholism', *Alcoholism Treatment Quarterly*, 20 (3–4), pp. 5–39. Available at: https://doi.org/10.1300/J020v20n03_02.

Leighton, T. (2017) *Inside the Black Box: An exploration of change mechanisms in drug and alcohol rehabilitation projects*. Bath: Bath University Press.

Leshner, A.I. (1997) 'Addiction is a brain disease, and it matters', *Science*, 278 (5335), pp. 45–47. Available at: https://doi.org/10.1126/science.278.5335.45.

Lewis, M.D. (2016) *The biology of desire: Why addiction is not a disease*. Melbourne and London: Scribe Publications.

Manning, E. (2013) *Always more than one: Individuation's dance*. Durham, NC: Duke University Press.

Manning, E. (2016) *The minor gesture*. Durham, NC: Duke University Press.

Marsh, T.N. et al. (2021) 'A study protocol for a quasi-experimental community trial evaluating the integration of indigenous healing practices and a harm reduction approach with principles of seeking safety in an indigenous residential treatment program in Northern Ontario', *Harm Reduction Journal*, 18(1), p. 35. Available at: https://doi.org/10.1186/s12954-021-00483-7.

Massumi, B. (2002) *Parables for the virtual: Movement, affect, sensation*. Durham, NC: Duke University Press.

Maté, G. (2013) *In the realm of hungry ghosts: Close encounters with addiction*. Mississauga, ON and London: Vintage Canada.

Maté, G. and Maté, D. (2022) *The myth of normal: Trauma, illness & healing in a toxic culture*. London: Vermilion.

Nicholson, H. (2014) *Applied drama: The gift of theatre*. 2nd ed. Basingstoke and New York: Palgrave Macmillan.

Ornell, F., Moura, H.F., Nichterwitz Scherer, J., Pechansky, F., Paim Kessler, F.H. and von Diemen, L. (2020) 'The COVID-19 pandemic and its impact on substance use: Implications for prevention and treatment', *Psychiatry Research*, 289, p. 113096. Available at: https://doi.org/10.1016/j.psychres.2020.113096.

Parkinson, C. (2015) 'The recoverist manifesto'. *Issuu*. Available at: https://issuu.com/artsforhealth/docs/rm_online_version (accessed 3 March 2018).

Schaef, A.W. (1987) *When society becomes an addict*. San Francisco, CA: HarperCollins.

Segal, G.M.A. (2014) *Twelve steps to psychological good health and serenity: A guide*. New York: Grosvenor House Publishing. Available at: http://public.eblib.com/choice/publicfullrecord.aspx?p=1685068 (accessed 1 November 2017).

Segal, G. (2017) 'How an addict's power of choice is lost and regained', in N. Heather and G. Segal (eds), *Addiction and choice: Rethinking the relationship*. Oxford and New York: Oxford University Press, pp. 365–384.

Shiner, M., Carre, Z., Delsol, R. and Eastwood, N. (2018) 'The colour of injustice: Race, drugs and law enforcement in England and Wales – a briefing paper'. London: StopWatch, Release, London School of Economics. Available at: https://www.release.org.uk/sites/default/files/pdf/publications/The%20Colour%20of%20Injustice.pdf (accessed 4 January 2019).

Sloan, C. (2014) 'From "Substance Misuse: The Musical" to "Double Whammy": The Affect of Outside Edge Theatre Company', in J. Reynolds and Z. Zontou (eds), *Addiction and Performance*. Newcastle upon Tyne: Cambridge Scholars Publishing, pp. 214–233.

Thompson, J. (2011) *Performance affects: Applied theatre and the end of effect*. Basingstoke and New York: Palgrave Macmillan.

1 Creating Spaces of Potentiality through Collaborative Theatre-Making

In September 2017, I presented *The Antidote* at the Collisions festival of practice research at the Royal Central School of Speech and Drama. This was a short, devised theatre piece created in collaboration with a group of performers with lived experience of recovery from addiction. Set within a dystopian future world, the narrative of the performance explored the interactions of a group of 'addicts' who were impounded in a holding room. The exchanges that occurred within this fictional confined space served as an attempt to convey the difficulties and complexities of maintaining recovery-orientated ways of being within a hostile environment. Comprising two women and three men aged 35–65 years, the group came from varied backgrounds, and included one South Asian person, one Irish person, and three people from working-class backgrounds; two members of the group had professional actor training. All self-identified as 'in recovery'. The characters they created for the performance were representative of experiences across a spectrum of addictions, specifically drugs, alcohol, sex and food, as well as mental illness.[1]

It seems fitting, in my attempts to capture the messy connections of recovery-engaged performance practice, to begin with a close analysis of my own approach which builds upon my prior experience as a practitioner with Outside Edge Theatre Company. How can I offer observations on the practice of others without first understanding my own processes and ethos? Subsequently, in this chapter and the next, I critically reflect on discoveries arising from my documentation of the collaborative theatre-making process involved in the making of *The Antidote*.[2] I had invited the five performers to participate alongside me in a research inquiry into the ways in which a recovery-engaged approach to theatre-making might influence the ethical and political priorities that orientate particular relational experiences during, and perhaps beyond, the collaborative process. The analysis of this practice experiment assists with relating the theoretical concepts of practice as an affective ecology to the discussion of a recovery-engaged orientation to performance-making. Observations are drawn from documentation recorded during the process, including audio and video recordings. In keeping with the approach to 'messy connections' discussed previously, I attend to the 'traces' of relation that linger in the documentation and that, if engaged

DOI: 10.4324/9781003271062-2

with, might stimulate new occasions of experience in the future (Manning 2016, 36).

A Space of Potentiality

I consider theatre-making to be a process of facilitating a *space of potentiality* which operates as a temporary environment in which participants might be enabled to make new discoveries through the energetic and sensorial activities used to create a performance collaboratively. To outline what I mean by this, I conceptualise the relational experience of theatre-making through philosophical concepts of the body, or the experience of being, as evolving through relation with its surroundings and space as a facilitated 'milieu' in which relation takes place.

My use of the term 'milieu' refers to the environment, or surroundings, in which being is in relation. One might think of it as the systems of connectivity, or relation that surround us. A milieu, drawing on philosopher Gilbert Simondon's interpretation of it, might be composed of the resonances of experience from different temporalities as well as including the bodies of different organisms and objects ([1958] 2016, 59). In this chapter, I use the term 'space of potentiality' to refer to the facilitated milieu of performance activity. This differs slightly from the milieu discussed by Simondon, and later Manning (2013), in that I acknowledge that there is a degree of intentionality on the part of the arts practitioner in priming a process that generates certain bodily and spatial relations for the purpose of making a performance.

Manning's interpretation of milieu as a constellation of bodies, human and nonhuman, is useful for transposing Simondon's concept to an analysis of performance practice and with the staging of bodies in performance (2013, 19). In particular, she discussed human existence as a complex ever-evolving system of relations fuelled by the affective capacities of the organic and in-organic forces in 'co-constellation' within a given environment (19). Furthermore, her concept of the body as an 'ecology of processes', propelled into movement by the affective sensation of relation with a given constellation assists in translating Simondon's notion of individuation (the process of becoming into being) to the activity of performance-making.

I draw from Manning's 'co-constellation' of bodies an indication of how the affective experience of theatrical performance might serve as a mechanism for exploring the ways in which bodies, identities and societal relations evolve. When analysing performance-making with people in recovery, I consider my collaborators to be bodies-in-process involved in navigating the affective dimensions of their experience of the world in order to develop a way of being that incorporates practices that support a recovery-orientated existence. Through application of philosophical concepts of being as in constant movement in response to encounters with others (Manning 2013, 16), I highlight the productive ways in which applied performance practice might intersect with the gradual change associated with recovery from addiction.

This understanding of performance practice as a relational experience is also founded upon my application of the concept of individuation to the experience of recovery from addiction. Manning's interpretation of Simondon's concept of individuation is especially poignant for developing a deep understanding of the existential dimension of recovery from addiction. For Simondon, individuation encapsulates the reaction that occurs when forms of being attempt to resolve the moment of instability generated through interaction with the constituents – human or nonhuman – of its surrounding environment ([1964] 1992, 302). Like individuation, a body in recovery is always unfinished, ever changing and responding to interactions with the surrounding systems of the world in which it inhabits. A practitioner working with people in recovery should, therefore, understand that recovery is an ongoing process and that performance activity might increase their capacity to engage in recovery processes. Conversely, inappropriate practice can hinder recovery.

Posthumanist approaches to addiction research have outlined the importance of developing a nuanced understanding of the contextual experiences of each event of 'using'[3] in addiction. In particular, Duff's concept of the drug assemblage highlighted that 'each event of consumption combines spaces, bodies, affects and relations in the expression of drug effects' (2014, 127). I expand this assemblage approach to all forms of addiction-based activity and consider the possibilities of theatrical performance in addressing the lived experience of addiction as a contextualised event that is influenced by a complex range of factors that differ according to the varying attributes of the addicted person and their surroundings. Recovery, according to Duff, is a process of navigating bodily and spatial connections that increase one's capacity for wellness (2016, 58). I consider Manning's philosophy to add to this discussion a conduit for also addressing the human psychobiology involved in recovery from addiction without essentialising the body. Drawing on Manning, I consider the body as a 'relational field' (2013, 19) within which the physical, neurological and psychosocial converge to become an individual's lived experience.

Manning's interpretation of individuation into movement illustrates each phase of being as a series of tendencies or inclinations that converge in a moment of experience, a transition point, similar to a dancer's bodily movement (2013, 16). I relate Manning's concept of human ecology to the experience of human connection, interaction and the embodied sensation of participation in theatre-making. Creating a performance might be considered as an ecology of processes of active engagement with one's surroundings, propelled into interaction through the embodied sensation of creative activity with others. My understanding of *affect* is framed within an ecology of being and a process of facilitating connection and interrelation that opens a space for potentiality to emerge.

Through applying both Manning's and Simondon's process philosophies to examine how affect operates as a force of being, experienced through relation with one's surroundings, I propose that the ethics of navigating change in recovery-engaged practice might be addressed through the participatory and

Creating Spaces of Potentiality through Collaborative Theatre-Making 23

ethical-political ethos of the arts practitioner and the participants who are positioned as collaborators. As O'Grady indicated, the practitioner must take account of their philosophical motivations in how navigations of openness, risk and vulnerability are managed through artistic, pedagogical and political commitments (2017, 13). By outlining what I consider to be a space of potentiality in the rest of this section, I reveal my ethical and political priorities in how I utilised a recovery-engaged approach to theatre-making.

While there were specific features of *The Antidote* process that were distinctly recovery-engaged, it is useful to note that my underpinning approach to facilitating the theatre-making activity also drew on principles of practice that feature across the field of applied theatre. My reflections in this chapter, therefore, focus upon the following themes that were not only relevant to my recovery-engaged practice, but also resonate with debates across applied theatre-making. First, *embracing potentiality* as an ethical and political commitment; second, *approaching space as plural, liminal and sensorial* in the context of theatre-making; and third, *facilitating dynamic and reflexive relations* among participants and with their surrounding context that support potentiality.

Embracing Potentiality

Day two of the series of devising workshops began with a check-in.[4] We sat in a circle in the performance room that was our base for the duration of the devising process and where the scratch performance would be shared with a public audience. Each member of the group was invited to share their thoughts and feelings on beginning the second day of creative activity. One member of the group, Adi, was absent due to illness. I was feeling a degree of nervousness and apprehension about this early stage of the process, concerned that Adi might be unable to continue and whether the group process would be productive. Counter to my internal concerns, the rest of the group shared comments that emphasised excitement, particularly a pleasure in anticipation of the new ideas or creative discoveries they expected would unfold that day. Sarah's comment, below, highlighted relation with the theatrical space.

> I really enjoyed yesterday. I really like being here. I just like the potential of it. It's just a black box and that's my favourite starting point, from absolutely nothing, a blank space. And I liked the exercise we did, the little thing with Adi where we began to explore the space … and to have the freedom to do that. It's nice … I like that, if I wanted to work under the table there, I could.
>
> (Day two of *The Antidote* workshops)

For Sarah, the performance space invoked exploration, potential and freedom in not knowing what the performance was yet to be. An emphasis on the potential, or indeterminate, discoveries of performance activity is also pertinent to my ethical commitments in a practice that works with people affected by addiction. This serves as a useful contrast to the notion of choice that has been equated to the dilemma of addiction. For instance, addiction as a 'willful choice' has been much discussed in the decades of addiction research (Heather and Segal 2017; Yaffe 2001; Levine 1985). Debate ranges across themes such as moral failing (Levine 1978), neurological dysfunction (Panksepp et al. 2002), epigenetic inheritance (Nestler 2014) and psychological akrasia (Heather 2017). Yet the lived experience of the apparent choice to perpetuate addiction-based activity is complicated by the force of a combination of surrounding factors that create the 'assemblage' of any event of 'using' (Duff 2014, 127). I consider, therefore, that any appreciation of recovery from addiction must also acknowledge the contextual and systemic features that reinforce addiction in how they hinder the development of capacities for recovery.

The issue of choice in addiction research and recovery approaches also correlates with the ethical dilemmas discussed in applied theatre around agency and transformation. Addiction therapist and recovery writer Ann Wilson Schaef considered recovery as a 'choice not to die' (1987, 16). Her assumption was that addiction eventually leads to death. I invoke Manning's use of ecology to consider people in recovery as bodies-in-process that are engaged in change through inter- and intrapersonal interaction. The practices of recovery adopted to support this development may be considered as a perpetual renewal of a choice 'not to die' in favour of developing an increased capacity to experience aliveness. I consider aliveness to be affective in how it operates as a force of desire to connect with others, with the surrounding environment and to experience *being* differently. Choice might, therefore, be reframed within the process of recovery as a desire for and commitment to change. Subsequently, a recovery-engaged theatre practice operates in parallel to ongoing processes of change.

The problematic assumptions about the concept of change or of transformation in particular have been much discussed in discourses of applied theatre, thereby troubling the inherent power dynamics involved in agendas for change (Hughes and Nicholson 2016, 4) as well as the instrumentalisation of applied theatre work that leads to an over-emphasis on 'effects' as opposed to the aesthetic experience (Thompson 2011, 6). Concurrently, the limits of such a 'theatre of good intentions' and the implications of white, western-privilege have been addressed (Snyder-Young 2013, 22). In an academic era in which concepts of post-modernity have created an 'incredulity towards metanarratives', recognition of fluidity and multiplicity have superseded claims to fixed knowledge or 'truth' (Lyotard 2005 [1979], xiv). Additionally, contemporary applied theatre research takes place within the 'post-normal' context of the second decade of the 21st century in which simultaneous crises – financial, environmental, security and more – have undermined assumptions about normality, and the 'hegemonic rule of the west' upon which previous research paradigms may have been founded (O'Connor and Anderson 2015, 9 and 10).

Embracing Ziauddin Sardar's identification of the key features of the post-normal world, Peter O'Connor and Michael Anderson examined 'complexity, chaos and contradictions' as approaches to current research in applied theatre that offer 'critical hope' as a way of moving beyond the paralysis of a world that seems 'too complex for even complex solutions' (9 and 12). It is, then, perhaps unsurprising that Hughes and Nicholson suggest that contemporary applied theatre practices are more appropriately conceptualised as ecologies in which relations are contingent to the particular dynamics and features of any given context (2016, 5).

Individuation, as interpreted by Manning, illustrates the experience of life as a series of moments of 'becoming' (2013, 16). To relate this concept to applied theatre-making, I use the term 'potentiality'. In the context of theatre practice, I consider potentiality to denote a state of becoming that can be facilitated by priming the context and modes of relation that might instigate it. This state, or phase of creating performance, alludes to the unknown or indeterminacy of any moment of relation from which new ideas, movements or actions may emerge. As Sarah's comment above indicates, the early stages of theatre-making are inherently informed by the experience of not yet knowing what the performance will become. It is useful, therefore, to examine what it means to embrace indeterminacy as not only a phase of the artistic process, but also as an ethical and political commitment.

To explain further the rationale of this point, it is useful to consider Massumi's interpretation of the concept of 'becoming' within affect theory. Specifically, Massumi made an important distinction between the words 'potentiality' and 'possibility', interpreting the word 'possible' to be 'back-formed' by preconceived expectations (2002, 9). It is what a thing can be said to be when 'on target' (9). By this, I consider him to mean that to explore what is possible is already framed by the limitations of what might be deemed acceptable in accordance with a preconceived 'norm' or value judgement. Within applied theatre practice, this might materialise, for example, as the criteria that must be met to fulfil expectations set by funders of a project. In the context of recovery-engaged practice, I also consider how limitations can be inadvertently imposed through pre-established notions of what it means to be in recovery and, furthermore, what society values as a productive citizen.

Here, Massumi's emphasis on potentiality as virtual in its state of in-betweenness or not-yetness (2002, 30), is somewhat useful to considering how performance activity might facilitate such moments of, to use Sarah's word, 'freedom.' Rather than pre-cognitive, however, I suggest that affect is non-conscious in that it always-already mediated (Anderson 2014, 13); a moment of potential which may or may not become conscious in the act of 'performance' or interrelation in a creative process. It is a point of indeterminacy, as participants engage in making choices inspired by their creative imagination. I consider, therefore, that indeterminacy encapsulates the relative freedom of an in-between state of not-yetness when devising theatre. This is key to enabling a freer form of what might emerge in the creative process. Facilitating a process that supports indeterminacy opens up a greater experience of new potentialities that simultaneously gives participants more freedom of choice, not just artistically, but also to re-imagine themselves and their relation with the world around them. Potentiality, in my use of the term, offers a way of orientating my approach to applied theatre practice that evades normativity based on hegemonic values and the imposition of neoliberal social impact agendas, particularly in relation to imposing upon people in recovery from addiction pre-set expectations of recovery. It opens the potential of exploring how *they* wish to be in the world, beyond addiction. As Sean reflected during a discussion about recovery that occurred during day three of *The Antidote* workshops, 'you're building up your recovery image, y'know, this is me … there are certain guidelines that you make up for yourself'.

Indeterminacy, however, should not be confused with an avoidance of planning or preparation, nor does it mean a rejection of prior identity representations or past experience. Rather, the creative process of theatre-making allows for indeterminacy and so may become a space *for* potentiality; a space that is future-orientated and concerned with creative encounter and experimentation that embraces life as an ongoing process, rather than a fixed location. As Zontou suggested in relation to the work of *Fallen Angels Dance Theatre*, performances with people in recovery are a platform for 'becoming' that is aligned to the process of 'becoming recovered' (2017, 217). By this, she was referring to the cyclical process in which people in recovery 'revisit their past experiences as a means of both reconciling their past with their present and finding ways to move forward' (217).

During *The Antidote* workshops, indeterminacy was embraced through the way in which the process of creating a performance was facilitated. As the facilitator, I was open to sharing responsibility, and therefore decision-making power, with my group of collaborators. On several occasions, during check-ins and informally during breaks, members of the group would share expressions of excitement and curiosity about what the performance might be. In particular, one member would arrive each morning with a new idea for his character. This, at times, posed dilemmas in how creative suggestions were negotiated and either included or not. Maintaining an openness to chance was not always a comfortable experience for me as the person with ultimate responsibility for the conduct of proceedings. Ultimately, I realised that what mattered was my – and the group's – approach to constructing spatial and bodily relations that embraced the at times uncomfortable uncertainty of potentiality. Theatrically, this was aided by the emphasis on improvisation as a devising strategy. During the check-in on day three of the workshops, I reflected with the group that in the course of the improvisation process I had felt a sense of creative flow when I had stopped thinking about what the performance should be and instead allowed the group to physically offer and explore ideas.

> I was able to forget about the anxiety of 'we need to have something' because I had forced myself to stop being a perfectionist, stop trying to

control things, just let be and go. And I think, in doing that, I allowed myself to be open to what would happen and I was offered what you threw at me, which was lots of fantastic and interesting moments that we can now work on and develop.

(Day three of *The Antidote* workshops)

Extending my reflection to the experience of recovery, I later shared during the check-out at the end of day three that perhaps theatrical improvisation is healing in that it forces those involved to 'be present', or what acting teachers might refer to as *being in the moment*. By being fully immersed in the moment of creative activity, anxieties or intrusive thoughts are pushed aside by bodily, sensory interaction within the facilitated space. Or, as Adi stated during the same check-out, 'Doctor drama, I think, it's made me feel a lot better' (day three of *The Antidote* workshops).

Approaching Space as Liminal, Plural and Sensorial

By space, I refer to the construction of a time-bound affective experience that can be facilitated by a theatre practitioner with those with whom they are creating a performance. Invariably, space is also connected to place. Drawing on contemporary research and theory on place (Mackey 2016; Massey 2005; Thrift 2008), I accept that a concept of place as a set defined entity does not correspond to the subjective experience of that place, especially when engaged in creative activity that encourages the participant to think beyond the geographical setting in which they are currently situated. In fact, Mackey's work on 'performing locations' has demonstrated how applied theatre practice can 'destabilise suppositions' about any given place (2016, 107). Using theatre practices to explore and interrogate participants' relations with a given place, such as the Performing Local Places Project, Mackey has shown how place is not static and is indeed bound up in relational experiences that may also change.[5]

This chapter does not interrogate relations with specific places, although I am mindful of the effect that the particular resonance of a place may have on the participants with whom I have worked. For instance, they may have certain drug-using memories associated with the location in which our rehearsal or performance venue is based.[6] Often the new experience of performing while clean and sober does allow participants to alter their relationship with this place. For the purpose of outlining the concept of a *space of potentiality*, I wish to focus on the relations and practices within the affective experience of a theatrical rehearsal or devising process. Massey's concept of space 'as process' is, therefore, relevant to the philosophical approach adopted in this book (2005, 11). She emphasised space as 'always under construction' through the relations that occur in a given place and moment (9). Her proposition that space as spheres of interrelation correlates with Manning's notion of milieu as a constellation, particularly in how Massey predicates this on the overlapping of plural and multiple possibilities (11). Space is a sphere in which different potentialities may coexist.

Space in the plural form, in that there is always more than one potential narrative or experience, is pertinent to the context of the experience of theatre-making with people in recovery. Creating any performance requires an openness to potential ideas, to a multiplicity of expressions through body and voice. Given the complex and varied experiences of addiction, performance practice with people in recovery from addiction should especially support the expression of multiple narratives of different experience. This requires facilitation of a plurality of expressions of lived experiences, histories, identities and aspirations that may emerge from any given group of participants. Each of my collaborators in *The Antidote* had their own unique addiction and recovery narratives that were marked by the ways in which their particular bodies-in-process were racialised, gendered or classed. Although they shared common values of being in recovery, their expressions of difference were also hugely valued and encouraged with the facilitated space.

To conceptualise the creation of such a space, I suggest that potentiality might be associated with the concept of liminality, now ubiquitous in performance studies. Liminality usefully correlates to the notion of becoming, or individuation, discussed in Chapter 2 in that I associate it with a state of in-betweenness. As Jon McKenzie noted, Richard Schechner's discussion of liminality provided performance theory with a model for 'theorising the transformative potential' of theatre and performance (2001, 36)[7]. Subsequently, performance scholars accepted the liminality of performance as 'spatial, temporal, and symbolic in-betweeness' (50). This indicates a temporal dimension, or perhaps a sense of in-between or suspended time that correlates with the discussion of becoming, or potentiality, mentioned earlier.

Recovery-engaged theatre practice, therefore, includes embodied experience that carries resonances from past experience as well as holding the potential for generating future experience. Time is not static, but is layered with the past, present and future. This was particularly evident when listening to the conversations among my collaborators that occurred during breaks and personal reflections that occurred outside of the process. For instance, Hannah and Sean shared humorous anecdotes about their past addictive behaviour, including a tale about sneaking out of hospital before surgery to grab a drink at the local pub with markings drawn on the cyst on their forehead that clearly demarcated the operation site – 'like a fucking unicorn'. These stories were included in the finished performance piece, although altered and anonymised, demonstrating how past experience can be folded into the creative process. Present reflections on recovery were also added to the piece, as will be shown in the following chapter. The facilitated creative process to which I subsequently refer as a space of potentiality conceives the theatrical space as also the 'coexistence of different temporalities' (Massey 2005, 40). This is particularly relevant when accounting for the complex psychobiology and sociopolitical aspects of the various context-specific experiences of addiction which one

Creating Spaces of Potentiality through Collaborative Theatre-Making 29

might encounter during recovery arts practice, as illustrated in the performance of *The Antidote*, that entail pasts, presents and potential futures.

In a review of the temporal dimension of her place practice, Mackey offered what I interpret as a repositioning of liminality to more explicitly address the experience of applied performance-making (2017, 11). She proposed that the experience of participation in performance activity generates an expansion or 'thickening of time' (11). By this she was referring to the slippage of feeling the passage of time through deep engagement with creative activity. Building upon her idea, I consider that a space of potentiality might operate as expanded, non-normative time. During *The Antidote* process, references were made by collaborators to slippage of time, but I suggest that the most poignant feature was the extended time devoted to reflections on experience of recovery through various modes of bodily expression that also allowed for an overlap of the resonances of previous, present and potential future experiences. This 'thickening' of time devoted to expression of recovery experience and interpersonal exploration indicates the recovery-engaged potential of non-normative time-spaces for people in recovery to discover and, perhaps, renegotiate changes in identity.

The implications of non-normative time for examining identity politics have already been discussed by prominent queer theorists. For instance, Elizabeth Freeman proposed the concept of 'chrononormativity' to reveal how time is manipulated by institutional structures of power through which lives are organised to 'maximise productivity' (2010, 3). Time might be conceived as a 'bind' (3) to values that compel conformity to patterns of usage of time, particularly regarding work, reproduction and cultural activities that reinforce a hetero-norm. Indeed, people affected by addiction are likely to have experienced a way of life outside of the usual organisational structures of work and family. The absorption of time through compulsive cycles of 'using' creates slippage from linear constructs of the passage of time.

Queer theory's suggestion of disruptions to time and monolithic notions of 'normal' are useful in demonstrating how the liminal space of performance practice might enable experiences that are non-normative. In particular, researchers of queer performance, such as Stephen Farrier (2015, 140) and Joe Parslow (2019, 84) have demonstrated how queer performance practices disrupt normative notions of time. The liminality of a theatrical time-space might, therefore, offer an experience counter to the pressures of conformity to a social norm beyond the facilitated space that, as noted earlier, hinder capacities for recovery by imposing value judgements upon lives that have been lived differently. A space of potentiality might then be conceived as a liminal milieu in which time is expanded, allowing extended inter-personal exploration on issues related to life experience, and also as non-normative in that it is cultivated by the people involved in the activity who may choose to explore their newly emerging identities in a space unfettered by prevailing societal expectations of what is considered to be normal.

A liminal milieu is also affective in that lived experience within it is sensorial; in human terms, it is felt. Check-in and check-out contributions from my collaborators mainly began with a comment on how they felt before and after the devising workshop. Words such as excited, happy, nervous, tired, indicated a felt experience relating to their mood on entering the process or after the creative interaction of the activities that day.

The sensorial aspect of performance activity has been discussed in the field of applied theatre, evident in the 'turn to affect' initiated by James Thompson, who argued in *Performance Affects: Applied Theatre and the End of Effect* that experiences of joy, fun, pleasure or beauty were the vital 'registry' of applied practice (2011, 116). The power of applied theatre is the affective impact of creating something beautiful, a 'moment of pleasurable, world-stopping sensation' experienced when watching or participating in artistic activity (140). It is an affect we feel an urge to share and so becomes political as it moves those who experience it towards engaging with others (144). Helen Nicholson has also emphasised the power of 'joyful encounters' in applied theatre that initiate a felt, collective experience (2014, 337). Both Thompson and Nicholson replace the concept of liminal with one of an affective encounter that is shared, whereby individual embodied experience is connected with others during the interrelation of the creation or sharing of a performance. Both liminality and affective sensation are features of a performance milieu in that liminality is the temporal dimension of the space in which it occurs and affect is the force of bodily sensation that fuels interrelation that generates the liminal moment.

Furthermore, I would suggest that the painful sensations of sadness, discomfort or anxiety are also important to the 'affective registry' of performance practice, particularly when working with people in recovery who are practising how to live with feelings and sensations that they have previously tried to avoid through drug or alcohol use or other compulsive behaviours. For instance, in conversation with my collaborators at the beginning of day three of the workshops, I reflected upon the way in which the performance project highlighted how the characters, and by association people in recovery, have confronted difficult aspects of their way of being in the world.

> We all have that dark side, but the uniqueness about the people in the 'tank' [the holding room setting of *The Antidote*] is that they have the unique experience of having to face that dark side and having to somehow negotiate forward. And it's not perfect, and not rosy, but there's a way of being in the world [in recovery] that becomes a willingness to challenge your own preconceived notions, catch yourself out when you're being judgemental, catch yourself out whenever you're dipping into that pain or anger or resentment, or all of those things.
> (Day three of *The Antidote* workshops)

Rather than framing the affective experience of performance as encounters of joy or pleasure, I consider such moments of creativity to be experiences of aliveness, capturing the wider gamut of Spinoza's 'affectus' that incorporates pleasure, pain and desire (1996, part III). Consequently, the *affect* – or feeling –

Creating Spaces of Potentiality through Collaborative Theatre-Making 31

of the creative encounter, is an embodied sensation of life. Spinoza's use of the word desire can subsequently be placed in the context of a will for life. To participate in making theatre may be a choice to feel alive through an affective experience in relation with others. It is a choice to share ideas, to reimagine and to experiment with new ways of being. For those in recovery from addiction, the choice to experience either pleasure or pain during performance comes from a desire to live, given that for many a continuation of active addiction would lead to eventual death. The renewed aliveness motivates connection, a desire to experience the world anew, that in turn generates moments of potentiality.

Such a sensorial space might, furthermore, be considered to generate the sensation of hope. Jill Dolan framed the affect of live performance as a utopic experience that generates a 'hopeful feeling' of what might be (2005, 2). To make claim to a utopic affect in applied theatre is, however, problematic and has been criticised. Selina Busby, in her critical evaluation of her decade-long applied theatre project in Dharavi, India (2006–2016), drew a distinction between utopic intentions that lead to abstract fantasy and the 'concrete utopia' or realisable achievement (2017, 99). In the case of her project, dreams of Bollywood stardom are contrasted with the real-life progress of the project's translator who becomes an applied theatre practitioner. Busby's concerns about concrete hope are relevant to applied performance with people in addiction recovery, particularly with regard to the precarity of recovery and, often, the socioeconomic challenges they face in pursuing artistic aspirations. Performance practice must not offer a 'cruel optimism' in the manner described by Lauren Berlant (2010, 369–370) through which hope, or desire, is attached to unrealisable promises of a better future. Indeed, cruel optimism resonates closely with the experience of active addiction, whereby an addicted person becomes gripped by their source of phantasmal promise despite injurious consequences. The risk of perpetuating cruel optimism in this work, promises of recovery or aspirational goals that may not be achievable, is all the more reason to shed fixed targets to define the personal change that may emerge from any given recovery arts project.

Positioning recovery arts practice as a positive addiction may, consequently, overlook the consequences of enabling attachments to a 'compromised' promise of a recovery 'high'. Rather than seeking replacement highs, I consider recovery as an effort towards balance through acquiring ways of being that nurture a less extreme response to life experience that feature in the compulsive patterns of addiction. Adi's comment, below, about addiction demonstrates this point.

> It's the nature of the mind, it gets attached to things … And I think that that's where a lot of addictions stem from because the mind wants to latch on to something and obsess about it. I'm obviously talking about substances 'cos many of us have come to this through that, but, as Sarah was saying earlier, you've got the whole wealth of addictions, like gambling

and young people these days with social media ... But I think it's about channelling it in the right ways and being aware of it and having that balance in life and making sure you give adequate time to all the important areas.

(Day one of *The Antidote* workshops)

Ultimately, the construct of space to which I refer in this chapter is founded upon the assumption, as discussed above, that it is facilitated through the patterns of relation with those assembled during the event of theatrical activity. While I extend this to discuss objects and place in Chapters 3 and 4, my focus below addresses the specifically human-to-human relations during the creative process.

Facilitating Dynamic and Reflexive Interactions

Much of what has been discussed so far relies on the way in which interaction during a collaborative creative process is facilitated. The ethos, or ethical and political values, of the facilitator of this experience is, therefore, a key influence on how interaction is instigated, guided and managed. Much has been written in the field of applied theatre of how such creative spaces are facilitated through modes of collaboration and ethos of practice, such as Nicholson's 'sensory pedagogy' (2014, 62) or Kathleen Gallagher's 'micro-politics' (2016, 233). My own ethos as an applied practitioner is founded, as far as is possible, on a non-hierarchical devising process that positions creative activity as a co-initiative from which there is joint ownership of the performance that emerges. This involves an openness to sharing control of the devising process with collaborators which challenges me to embrace the relative risk of indeterminacy. As O'Grady proposed, 'exploring the unknown' is essential to a creative process (2017, viii–ix) which, consequently, requires commitment to a 'radical openness' that embraces the indeterminacy of not knowing (11). Such openness to chance, especially within the context of my own practice, often accepts 'critical vulnerability' (2) as an aesthetic choice through which trust, risk and psychological safety are negotiated.

In the example of *The Antidote*, the construction of a 'safe' and 'open' space for creative exploration was aided by the fact that the performers who agreed to take part in the research workshops had worked with me before. This meant that the process began with a shared understanding of my approach to creative collaboration upon which we could develop. Given that a certain level of trust, and relations of care, were pre-established, the creative exploration of the chosen theme, 'Recovery', began with a greater degree of openness and willingness to experiment than may have been possible with an unfamiliar group. Furthermore, this group had significant experience of recovery, considerable 'clean time', in that they had each been engaged in programmes of recovery for several years, even decades. Consequently, they could be considered to have greater resilience in their recovery compared to people in the early stages of a recovery process. I appreciate, therefore, that this example of practice was contingent on the extensive recovery experiences of those involved.

Concepts of 'safe space' and participant 'agency' have been debated (Hunter 2008; Prendergast and Saxton 2010; White 2013) and there is a general acceptance that an ethically aware arts practitioner must consider issues relating to safety, either physical or psychological, and, as Hughes and Nicholson stated, the inextricable power dynamics inherent in theatre-making (2016, 4). I am specifically interested in how a practice of recovery from addiction may generate a particular approach to navigating interactions and power dynamics. I will elaborate further on the recovery-engaged forms of reflection in the chapter that follows. Here, I focus on what a recovery-orientated ethics might be in this work. Much of the early stage of addiction recovery involves learning – or relearning – new ways of interacting with oneself and the surrounding world. Consequently, it requires a willingness to not only identify unhelpful thinking and behavioural patterns but also to develop new ways of perceiving and interacting. These patterns were evident in some of the comments shared during *The Antidote* workshops. For instance, Adi's comment in response to a debate among the group illustrates the reflexive process of a recovery practice.

> 'Cos, y'know, I did the SMART recovery stuff and we talk about irrational beliefs we carry, and disputing these irrational beliefs – and even if it might be true, what's the healthiest thing for you is to think of the most magnanimous thing, rather than the suspicious addict part of your brain.
> (Day four of *The Antidote* workshops)

Nigel Thrift's concept of an ethics of *out-of-jointness* especially resonates with my understanding of the reflexive mindset of recovery, as shown by Adi above. By adopting an orientation towards out-of-jointness, by making the familiar strange, he proposed an approach that embraced creating a new experience of life, of oneself, a letting go of what you think you know (Thrift 2008, 14). I propose, therefore, an ethics of out-of-jointness in performance practice that supports dynamic and reflexive interactions through a commitment to challenge all involved, including the theatre practitioner, to look anew at what they think they know and so allow a space for potentiality to emerge. Fusing this with creative activity that invites novelty and explores new expressions of what it means to be in the world, be that through body or voice, allows 'newness' to become into being which opens up a space for potentiality to flourish. Thrift referred to a 'boosting aliveness' by moving beyond the limits we inhabit in everyday life through a concern with the future, which also opens up to hope (2008, 15).

During *The Antidote* workshops, my application of these ethics was evident in my approach to negotiating co-creation and the monitoring of my personal responses to the process. Initially, in the role of facilitator, I guided warm-up exercises and set up stimuli or provocations for creative exploration. As the process unfolded and we began to discuss, reflect on and develop the characters and content for a performance, I assumed the role of mediator in the collaborative process. Each collaborator took responsibility for inventing and developing their chosen character. I focused on assisting the negotiation of their creative contributions to reach a loose consensus of ideas that could be performed. An openness to exploring suggestions that I did not personally like or thought would not work was crucial to support the willingness expressed by the group to experiment with everyone's creative ideas. This required, on my part, a willingness to share power with – and even relinquish to – the group during the devising process. The exchange below offers what I consider to be a comical example of my practice of reflexivity and acceptance in a moment during which I chose to relinquish power and accept the flow of chaos:

ME: Let's do one more run-through before we finish today.
DAVE: Shall I dim the lights? (*He walks towards the main light switches on the wall of the studio room*)
ME: No thanks. Those lights take a long time to turn back on. They're ...
DAVE: I'll turn off this one. (*He flicks a switch and half the room becomes dark*).
ME: It's better just to leave them on.
SARAH: Dave, just leave it.
DAVE: (*He flicks the lighting switch back on, but the lights don't respond. He turns the other switches off and on, but the lights don't respond immediately*) Oh, the lights won't come on.
SARAH: Dave!
ME: (*Releasing a chuckle and sigh*) (*We stand in the dim light of the darkened room, waiting for the lighting lamps to slowly regain power*).
(Day four of *The Antidote* Workshops)

On reflection, the moment above indicated to me the instances when I was challenged to accept the chaos that can occur when one hands over control of a process to others. I did not insist on holding supreme authority or on compliance to my instructions as other theatre directors might, although I held a position of leadership within the group that I could use if desired or necessary.[8] This was an ethico-political decision on my part, as I knew from my previous work that many people in recovery have past experiences of transgressing societal 'rules'. As indicated earlier, recovery entails the acquisition of skills to modulate former impulsive tendencies and I consider this skill to require a level of agency and accountability that would not be nurtured by dominant leadership styles. The test for me, during the moment above, was to transfer my feeling of frustration into a calmer, perhaps more balanced, acceptance that the run-through would be delayed while we waited for Dave to stop fiddling with the lights.

Conclusion

The conditions discussed throughout this chapter form the basis of an understanding of what I consider to be a space of potentiality in applied performance practice. I propose this as an ethico-political engagement with the process of facilitating a liminal milieu (a non-normative expanded time-space) through modes of relation with bodies, space and, consequently, time. Within the context of working with people in recovery, this concept reframes discussions about change and affect to conceptualise recovery as a process of regeneration through interrelation with one's surroundings that increase capacity for 'becoming well' (Duff 2016, 58). Embracing indeterminacy, or potentiality, that is supported by an 'ethics of out-of-jointness' (Thrift 2008, 14), can offer an experience counter to conventional societal values that might inhibit people with non-normative life experiences from discovering a recovery identity that works for them.

By embracing indeterminacy and the dynamic and reflexive interactions discussed above a space of potentiality is offered as a flexible and pluralist construct that is capable of responding organically to the variation of bodies, experiences and sensations that constellate within facilitated performance activity with people affected by addiction. The ethos described in this chapter assists in the facilitation of a space in which ideas of change or recovery identity can be explored free from the imposition of judgement, stigma and the associated affect of shame. Change might, instead, be conceived as the nurture of indeterminate regeneration. While such change within this conceptual framework does not conform to a set of criteria for success, I argue that the ethos described throughout this chapter assists a desire for connection with others, human and nonhuman, that in turn enhances capacity for recovery.

Notes

1 I refer to mental illness, here, as distinct from addiction. Addiction might be considered as an issue related to health and wellbeing; in this book, however, I recognise specific mental illnesses as separate. People affected by addiction may also have a diagnosis of a mental illness, often referred to in treatment services as a 'dual diagnosis'. My collaborators chose to include specific mental illnesses in *The Antidote* to represent their own knowledge and understanding of living with dual diagnosis.
2 My collaborators have granted permission for their contributions to be shared. I have altered names to protect anonymity given the candidness of some of their comments.
3 The word 'using' is stated here in keeping with familiar recovery community parlance that denotes any addiction-based activity as using. This is often equated to the consumption of substances; however, I have often heard the word used to denote any activity that someone might be deemed addicted to – for instance, 'using' food or 'using' pornography.
4 In this style of practice a check-in operates in a similar way to recovery group meetings in that each person takes turns to share their current thoughts or feelings. Each person in the group may share without interruption or subsequent comment from the group to maintain a non-judgemental and non-controlling dynamic. In my

practice, I initiate the process as the facilitator and director by beginning with my own reflection that models an emphasis on my personal reflections on the creative activity and feelings that arise from it. This establishes a difference between a recovery meeting and a theatre-making process, while enabling collaborators to acknowledge and process recovery-related sensations where necessary.
5 The Performing Local Places project took place in Camden and Oldham (2016–2017) using arts practices to develop 'place attachment' to promote community wellbeing with two particular communities, those affected by homelessness (Camden) and new migrants (Oldham). See http://www.performingplaces.org/docs/ppbrochure.pdf (accessed 18 April 2017).
6 When travelling with members of Outside Edge Theatre to perform a show, one performer pointed out local streets and shared memories of 'grafting' for money and scoring heroin.
7 Marvin Carlson contributed further to the application of liminality to performance studies by emphasising that liminal in performance equates to anti-structure, transgressing the normal structure of cultural operations (2004, 18). For Carlson, performance, especially the playful and reflexive aspects of theatrical performance activity, becomes a 'special laboratory for cultural negotiations' (214).
8 My caveat here is that I hold responsibility for the physical and psychological wellbeing of the group and, should that be placed at risk by a member of the group, I deem it my responsibility to use my position of leadership to deal with the issue as appropriately as the context allows. For instance, in a previous context with a different group, a colleague and I asked a member to leave because they made threats of violence to others in the group.

References

Anderson, B. (2014) *Encountering affect: Capacities, apparatuses, conditions.* Farnham and Burlington, VT: Ashgate.
Berlant, L. (2010) 'Cruel optimism', in M. Gregg and G.J. Seigworth (eds), *The affect theory reader.* Durham, NC: Duke University Press, pp. 94–117.
Busby, S. (2017) 'Finding a concrete utopia in the dystopia of a "sub-city"', *Research in Drama Education: The Journal of Applied Theatre and Performance*, 22 (1), pp. 92–103. Available at: https://doi.org/10.1080/13569783.2016.1263557.
Carlson, M. (2004) *Performance: A critical introduction.* 2nd ed. New York: Routledge.
Dolan, J. (2005) *Utopia in performance: Finding hope at the theater.* Ann Arbor: University of Michigan Press.
Duff, C. (2014) *Assemblages of health: Deleuze's empiricism and the ethology of life.* New York: Springer.
Duff, C. (2016) 'Atmospheres of recovery: Assemblages of health', *Environment and Planning A*, 48 (1), pp. 58–74. Available at: https://doi.org/10.1177/0308518X15603222.
Farrier, S. (2015) 'Playing with time: Gay intergenerational performance work and the productive possibilities of queer temporalities', *Journal of Homosexuality*, 62 (10), pp. 1398–1418. Available at: https://doi.org/10.1080/00918369.2015.1061361.
Freeman, E. (2010) *Time binds: Queer temporalities, queer histories.* Durham, NC: Duke University Press.
Gallagher, K. (2016) 'The micro-political and the socio-structural in applied theatre with homeless youth', in J. Hughes and H. Nicholson (eds), *Critical perspectives on applied theatre.* Cambridge and New York: Cambridge University Press, pp. 230–248.
Gordon, R. (2006) *The purpose of playing: Modern acting theories in perspective.* Ann Arbor: University of Michigan Press.

Heather, N. (2017) 'Addiction as a form of akrasia', in N. Heather and G. Segal (eds), *Addiction and choice: Rethinking the relationship*. 1st ed. New York: Oxford University Press, pp. 134–152.

Heather, N. and Segal, G. (eds) (2017) *Addiction and choice: Rethinking the relationship*. 1st ed. Oxford and New York: Oxford University Press.

Hughes, J. and Nicholson, H. (eds) (2016) *Critical perspectives on applied theatre*. Cambridge and New York: Cambridge University Press.

Hunter, M.A. (2008) 'Cultivating the art of safe space', *Research in Drama Education: The Journal of Applied Theatre and Performance*, 13 (1), pp. 5–21. Available at: https://doi.org/10.1080/13569780701825195.

Levine, H. (1985) 'The discovery of addiction: Changing conceptions of habitual drunkenness in America', *Journal of Substance Abuse Treatment*, 2 (1), pp. 43–57. Available at: https://doi.org/10.1016/0740-5472(85)90022-4.

Lyotard, J.-F. (2005) *The postmodern condition: A report on knowledge*. Repr. Manchester: Manchester University Press.

Mackey, S. (2016) 'Performing location: Place and applied theatre', in J. Hughes and H. Nicholson (eds), *Critical perspectives on applied theatre*. Cambridge and New York: Cambridge University Press, pp. 107–122.

Manning, E. (2013) *Always more than one: Individuation's dance*. Durham, NC: Duke University Press.

Manning, E. (2016) *The minor gesture*. Durham, NC: Duke University Press.

Massey, D.B. (2005) *For space*. London and Thousand Oaks, CA: SAGE.

Massumi, B. (2002) *Parables for the virtual: Movement, affect, sensation*. Durham, NC: Duke University Press.

McKenzie, J. (2001) *Perform or else: From discipline to performance*. London and New York: Routledge.

Nestler, E.J. (2014) 'Epigenetic mechanisms of drug addiction', *Neuropharmacology*, 76, pp. 259–268. Available at: https://doi.org/10.1016/j.neuropharm.2013.04.004.

Nicholson, H. (2014) *Applied drama: The gift of theatre*. 2nd ed. Basingstoke and New York: Palgrave Macmillan.

O'Connor, P. and Anderson, M. (2015) *Applied theatre. Research: Radical departures*. London: Bloomsbury.

O'Grady, A. (ed.) (2017) *Risk, participation, and performance practice*. New York: Palgrave Macmillan.

Panksepp, J., Knutson, B. and Burgdorf, J. (2002) 'The role of brain emotional systems in addictions: A neuro-evolutionary perspective and new "self-report" animal model', *Addiction*, 97 (4), pp. 459–469.

Parslow, J. (2019) 'Come hear the music play: The politics of queer failure and practices of survival', in T. Fisher and E. Katsouraki (eds), *Beyond failure: New essays on the cultural history of failure in theatre and performance*. London: Taylor & Francis, pp. 80–94.

Prendergast, M. and Saxton, J. (2010) *Applied theatre: International case studies and challenges for practice*. Bristol and Chicago: University of Chicago Press.

Schaef, A.W. (1987) *When society becomes an addict*. San Francisco, CA: HarperCollins.

Simondon, G. (1992) 'The genesis of the individual', in J. Crary and S. Kwinter (eds), *Incorporations*. 1st ed. New York: Zone, pp. 297–319.

Simondon, G. (2016) *On the mode of existence of technical objects*. Minneapolis, MN: Univocal Publishing.

Snyder-Young, D. (2013) *Theatre of good intentions: Challenges and hopes for theatre and social change*. London: Palgrave Macmillan. Available at: https://link.springer.com/openurl?genre=book&isbn=978-1-349-45104-3 (accessed 13 June 2018).

Spinoza, B.de (1996) *Ethics*. S. Hampshire and E.M. Curley (eds). London and New York: Penguin.

Thompson, J. (2011) *Performance affects: Applied theatre and the end of effect*. Basingstoke and New York: Palgrave Macmillan.

Thrift, N.J. (2008) *Non-representational theory: Space, politics, affect*. Abingdon and New York: Routledge.

White, G. (2013) *Audience participation in theatre: Aesthetics of the invitation*. Basingstoke and New York: Palgrave Macmillan.

Yaffe, G. (2001) 'Recent work on addiction and responsible agency', *Philosophy & Public Affairs*, 30 (2), pp. 178–221. Available at: https://doi.org/10.1111/j.1088-4963.2001.00178.x.

Zontou, Z. (2017) 'Upon awakening: Addiction, performance, and aesthetics of authenticity', in A. O'Grady (ed.), *Risk, participation, and performance practice: Critical vulnerabilities in a precarious world*. New York: Palgrave Macmillan, pp. 205–231.

2 Facilitating Recovery-Engaged Performance Atmospheres

It's February 2017, and I'm lying on the floor of the Wickham Theatre in Bristol, UK. The floor is cold, the room is in darkness except for the dim wash of yellow-orange light upon the central area of the room where FK Alexander sits on a tapestry cloth surrounded by an array of Tibetan singing bowls. A large screen displays digital images of microbial movement. To the right, two noise DJs stand behind a mixing desk. I'm a little confused. I feel the foam surface of the earplugs in my hand that were offered to me from a bowl held by the friendly usher at the entrance of the theatre when I walked in. What will I be needing these for? I close my eyes, as invited to do, and breathe deeply as I begin to feel the vibrations of sound move through the floor, through the air, through my body.

FK Alexander's performance of *Recovery*, which I experienced during the In-between Time international festival of performance art in Bristol 2017, generated a 'sonic milieu' (Gallagher 2016, 44) that was infused with an understanding of lived experience of addiction recovery. In the previous chapter I reflected on how human bodies might generate a temporary, liminal milieu through their interactions within a facilitated space-time. While I will continue the discussion of this and how the creative process of *The Antidote* created a specifically recovery-engaged milieu through interaction with peers in recovery, I also extend this thinking beyond the human to consider how a performance conducted largely through the sounds and vibrations of resonating objects can also generate a milieu that reminds us of the more-than-human features of addiction and recovery.

The milieu I refer to here is a 'constellation' of bodies, human and nonhuman, in which these constituents are in perpetual affective interrelation (Manning 2013, 19), creating a felt atmosphere. Both the collaborative creative process and the resultant staging of performance work generate constellations, some of the features of which might be intentionally primed to stage a story. Theses performance-based milieus are inherently unpredictable and cross-temporal. In this chapter, I proffer two features of milieu that relate productively to the experience of recovery-engaged performance. These features incorporate modes of interrelation experienced during recovery that also map onto the examples of performance practice shared in this chapter and throughout the book, namely *attunement* and *antagonism*.

DOI: 10.4324/9781003271062-3

Manning's reference to the milieu as a constellation conceptualises it as a relational field of 'affective attunement' (2013, 26). Specifically, she emphasised the experience of identity as constructed through relation with one's surroundings at any given moment (17). A constellation approach to understanding identity as composed of interactions within a particular environment assists with examining the ways in which people in recovery have been impacted, or defined by, interactions associated with addiction in their lives. This is particularly relevant for acknowledging how an 'addict' identity emerges in relation to the sociopolitical environment that includes systems of addiction treatment, criminal justice, media and entertainment that convey certain hegemonic values that inform what constitutes an 'addict'. Apply the additional intersections of race, gender, sexuality, disability and class and it becomes clear that there is a wide spectrum of nuanced judgements and discriminations that constitute differing experiences of 'addict' identities.

Ahmed's 'affective economies' highlight how societal norms and hierarchies are reinforced by the ways in which negative *affects*, such as hate or disgust, are projected upon – and stick to –certain bodies (2014, 8 and 12). In *The Cultural Politics of Emotion* (2014), Ahmed developed this argument to demonstrate how the bodies of black, Asian or minority ethnicities, particularly the feminine ones, become objects of hate or disgust in how their presence disrupts social hierarchies founded on male whiteness (4 and 58). Any discussion of milieu must, consequently, acknowledge the compromised attunements caused by past legacies of human-centred constructs of sociopolitical order. Perhaps, then, recovery-engaged performance can offer the potentiality of alternative attunements that might support the ongoing development of recovery identity?

Nonetheless, antagonism is an inherent feature of any environment. For Manning, coming into contact with difference is antagonistic to a static perception of our own identity (2007, 108). It disorientates what we think we know about ourselves. Antagonism or conflict, difference and disagreement, are essential features of the learning process. Without encounters with something, or somebody, that are different to what we already know about the world or ourselves, personal development is unlikely. Collaborative theatre-making is a particularly useful process for embracing difference and conflict. These attributes inform the making of new discoveries during creative performance activity as well as contributing to the generation of work that explores the tensions of 'becoming well' amid societal contexts that can inhibit bodily capacity for recovery. Theatrical or other modes of interdisciplinary performance can disrupt preconceived perceptions and challenge our prior attunements.

Attunement

It is day four of *The Antidote* workshops. The final workshop has finished and we are sitting in a circle, as we have done at the beginning and end of every session, each taking turns to share our thoughts, feelings or reflections on the experience of the workshop process. We have completed a full run-through of *The Antidote*. Sean begins and highlights a moment shared immediately after the performance. This moment is visibly registered as a shared facial expression, a smile, although the comments shown below reveal what I consider to be a more complex affective relation that instigated it,

SEAN: Yeah. I seen that smile on yer face earlier on, just now when you said 'that's it'. You seemed to be reasonably happy with what we've got so far. Which is great ... I'm happy with it.
ME: Thank you.
HANNAH: I've really enjoyed seeing you, all of you, for four days – and that smile [points to me], I remember that smile [others make sounds of agreement].

(Day four of *The Antidote* workshops)

Hannah's comment, in particular, reveals the significance of the moment for her in how she connects it to previous experience, a time before, and acquired knowledge from past creative collaboration with me and the group. Both comments reveal familiarity and somatic connection. Their chosen words are indicative of pleasure, specifically a sense of satisfaction in having achieved the collective goal of the performance task.

While Thompson (2011, 140) and Nicholson (2014, 337) have already discussed the significance of the 'joyful encounter' in creating applied theatre performance, I suggest here that the emotive expression shared above revealed a form of relation or connection akin to Manning's discussion of 'attunement' (2013, 26).

In particular, this moment highlighted, for me, the depth of connection established between myself and the group during the process of the workshops. As a practitioner, I was interested in tracing how this attunement operated during the creative process and how it was facilitated. Specifically, how interaction within the group and facilitated space created a recovery-engaged ethos. Heightened by the embodied knowledge of those in the space, processes of relation with others and societal context operated in uniquely recovery-infused ways.

Tuning into a Reflexive Process

To explain further, I propose that a distinct form of attunement operated through the group's bodily responses to the shared understanding of practices of recovery and the particular orientation towards their surroundings that this generated. Specifically, there was an increased level of self-awareness that also enhanced affinity with the others in the group. This revealed itself particularly during the check-in reflections. For instance, during the check-in on day one, a collaborator shared their thoughts before arriving at the workshop venue:

SARAH: My first thought is always alcoholic, it doesn't matter how long I've been in recovery, my first response to anything is alcoholic and I've learnt to get rid of the first thought. It's like pancakes, y'know, the first one goes in the bin. And so, my first thought is, 'Everyone will hate me, I don't fit in and Cathy's asked me because she feels sorry for me, or something, or she's run out of people to ask' [*she and I chuckle*] and I just have to say that and I know it's not true. Although I know it, the thought still comes. I think if I just put it out there, that's dumped ... And I'll feel more comfortable in the space.

(Day one of *The Antidote* workshops)

Sarah's comment revealed her awareness of the sensations she feels and how she experiences them as negative thoughts. She applied her experience of self-reflective practices of recovery to identify what she was feeling, but also acknowledged how this can impact on her perception of the intentions of others which might, in turn, influence her behaviour towards them. In the following comment, another collaborator stated,

SEAN: This morning I was leaving my flat ... and I got a little feeling, a little umph, and that umph I also got anytime we were going out to do a performance ... it's just a oooh [*claps hands, shivers shoulders – others murmur agreement*].

(Day one of *The Antidote* workshops)

Sean's comment also revealed an awareness of bodily sensations, but, in contrast to Sarah, it was a pleasurable sensation that we might interpret as excitement. Both comments are evidence that reflections were founded on a commitment to honesty about, and accountability for, personal bodily sensations.

Recovery practices require a particular ethic of reflexivity that is simultaneously supportive, respectful and challenging. When working with people in recovery, avoidance of the potential discomfort of critical reflection would be counterproductive to a recovery process that often entails a continual 'inventory' of thoughts and actions to encourage recognition of, and accountability for, addiction-orientated behaviour. This may also involve a recognition of thinking patterns or painful sensations of feeling that might inhibit relation with others, and also recovery. Relation in this context involves continual acts of reflexivity that support those involved to be open to relating with others while also practicing personal accountability. Sarah and Sean's comments above indicate some of the self-aware and reflexive practices of recovery. Expressions made by collaborators during check-ins throughout the creative process also revealed reflexive thinking about personal responses to the process and their capacity to affect others was apparent. For instance, on the first day (a Monday) Adi demonstrated a keen awareness of his own thinking patterns and his commitment to identifying how they link to addictive tendencies.

> Being back to work I've got into this thing of 'I hate Mondays', so I'm feeling a bit of lack of energy … But I'm really glad to be back in this kind of environment and it's taking me a bit of a while to get my mind set towards it … And with being off work this week, I'm still thinking about it and it takes me a few days just to get into another one. And I think that that's where a lot of addictions stem from because the mind wants to kind of latch on to something and obsess about it.
> (Day one of *The Antidote* workshops)

Performance practice, such as *The Antidote*, that uses reflexive practices that inevitably contain the memory of, or ongoing struggle with, personal experiences related to addiction risks the emergence of emotive and painful sensations. Recovery practices often entail learning how to cope with difficult feelings rather than avoiding them through addiction-based responses. During the process of working with my collaborators, I was mindful of my responsibility, as a practitioner, to be attuned to them and responsive to bodily and linguistic indications of discomfort too. Zontou has discussed the complex tension between vulnerable lives and risky aesthetics in the work of Fallen Angels Dance Theatre that uses autobiographical experience of addiction in their performances (2017, 211). Her discussion indicated that those involved in practice with people in recovery should 'problematise' the tension between the exposure caused through performing past experience and the potential empowerment of biographical performance (210).

During my previous practice with Outside Edge Theatre Company, we continually negotiated boundaries for respectful and inclusive interrelation, including the level of exposure that participants consented to experience in creative sharing or critical reflection. This was, on some occasions, uncomfortable and challenging. In particular, some participants, especially those in 'early' recovery from addiction, experienced fear and vulnerability more acutely. This is reflected in some of the comments cited from *The Antidote* workshops later in this section. Often, having used addictive behaviour, especially substances, to avoid painful feelings, processes of recovery involve learning to feel the intensity of emotion arising from past psychosocial experience, possibly including childhood difficulties or traumatic events.

The bodily sensation of shame is a particular affect that may impinge on the capacity for recovery and participation in collaborative arts activity. Although *The Antidote* collaborators were perhaps less hindered by sensations of shame than they might have been in earlier stages of their recovery, Sarah's comment, noted earlier, about her first 'alcoholic thought' indicates how shame is present as an ongoing sensation. Given that addiction functions as a codependent relationship and codependency is a condition considered to be founded on sensations of shame (or feeling 'less than worthy') it is useful to discuss briefly how performance practice might intervene with this sensation. I suggest intervention here with the view that shame can inhibit capacity for attunement with others and, consequently, restrict participation in performance and also recovery.

Brené Brown identified shame as a barrier to creativity, in that it fuels a fear of ridicule or the pain of being seen as unworthy which manifests into a reluctance to share creative ideas with others (2012, 185). Brown suggested that the paradox of shame is that it is also, ultimately, a fear of disconnection. Yet it is also a *cause* of disconnection because of the avoidant behaviour patterns a person might use to avoid feeling the pain of shame (2012, 68 and 77). Previously, cultural theorists Eve Kosofsky Sedgwick and Adam Frank drew upon Tomkins' theory of affect to consider shame as a paradoxical push away and pull towards sociability. With reference to queer identity, they demonstrated that the 'exquisite painfulness' felt in the social performance of shame becomes ingrained in self-identity (2003, 37). Considering identity as constructed through relation with one's surroundings, they considered that, for some, such relational encounters are imbued with painful experiences of shame and consequently their identity becomes marked by it (37). Their discussion of shame is useful to the discussion of practice in this chapter in that they proposed that shame should be embraced as part of the formation of certain experiences of identity (63). Through playing with the performativity of identity, they highlighted the possibilities of metamorphosed, reframed and refigured shame.

If shame operates through social performance, then perhaps recovery-engaged theatrical performance can offer people in recovery an opportunity for experimentation with different performances of identity. Consequently, through performance activity, they may renegotiate or re-navigate interrelation with others, to explore a different way of being, one beyond their current painful experience. Applying Manning's concept of constellations to theatre-making, therefore, offers a consideration of performance as an opportunity for generating a different milieu from the hegemonic norm in that it is informed by the bodily relations of collaborators who embody a different, recovery-orientated, world view. This is not only possible through the theatrical performance itself, but also occurs in the way in which relations with others in the group, including the facilitator, are navigated throughout the devising process. Creating a space for potentiality with people in recovery from addiction involves, therefore, an appreciation of vulnerability within the group and the corresponding modulations of shame felt by participants. I suggest that this occurred in *The Antidote* project through a shared attunement to the experiences of each member of the group that was supported by an understanding of recovery practices and perspectives. Such attunement also emanates from a mutual appreciation that vulnerability and perhaps painful, or uncomfortable, sensations are part of the process. Dave's comment at the end of the first workshop illustrates the point that this performance practice occurs alongside pain and discomfort.

> As I was coming down here, I was thinking I'll feel better when I'm here and interacting with other people ... 'Cos I have a lot of fear around getting ill. And doing these sorts of things [the performance workshops] is always a worry. Am I going to be OK? And, of course, I'd a bad night last night because there was a certain amount of preoccupation about that ... My worry is always whether physically wise I can keep the energy.
>
> (Day one of *The Antidote* workshops)

During the devising of *The Antidote*, all the collaborators demonstrated a willingness to share their reflections, enhanced, I suggest, by the relative safety of a space shared with others with similar recovery commitments. There were also responses from members of the group that indicated an affective relation to the reflections shared by others that I consider revealed a shared understanding of and an attunement to each other's recovery-orientated reflections. These reflexive responses occurred throughout the process, including the in-between moments of breaks, lunchtimes and even overnight. Often the content of their comments would shift across time and context. For instance, someone would share an idea for developing the performance, then add reflection on their own past experiences or literature they had read or a perspective on current events in the UK or world politics. Others would join in, adding their own perspectives on politics, society or past experiences. This indicated a cross-temporality to the affective relations that emerged in the creative space in that at any given moment there might be a simultaneity of bodily sensations invoked from memories, current events or musing about future aspirations. Listening to their conversations, I realised that the milieu of the creative activity was neither time-bound nor constrained to the theatrical space, the resonances of which lingered with the bodies involved.

As shown above, understanding recovery from addiction added a specific dimension to the processes of reflexivity, demonstrated through the collaborators' awareness of bodily sensations and how they affect thinking, behaving and relation with others. Such self-awareness is not necessarily exclusive to people in recovery, but, in this context, it revealed commitment to attuning oneself to the affective sensations of the body in order to find a sense of equilibrium through which it was possible to be receptive to others and the surrounding environment. I conceive such attunement as a crucial strategy for relapse prevention, whereby maintaining recovery requires an ability to monitor the potentially negative affect of relation with people, places or objects that might trigger former addictive responses. This is why I consider recovery to be an ongoing process of active and embodied learning. Patterns of reflexivity among the group revealed an acknowledgement of each other as people engaged in the ongoing process of recovery, as well as involved in a temporary theatre-making activity.

This reinforces the point made earlier that a practice of reflexivity that is simultaneously supportive, respectful and challenging is crucial. I also suggest that to attune to this manner of reflexivity in a theatre-making experience requires the practitioner to commit to, and indeed have the personal capacity to engage in, honest self-awareness and appraisal of their own behaviour and an openness to share some of this self-reflection. This might require a readjustment of personal boundaries for the practitioner, as well as a willingness to be critically reflexive about how one's own relative privilege, unconscious bias or previous experience might impact on affective attunement with participants or collaborators.

The embodied responses to creative stimuli were distinctive in their connection to a shared understanding of survival, a working through painful lived experience. This was evident in movement montages created on the theme of recovery as well as improvised scenes. For instance, in response to a stimulus of music by an artist in recovery, the group created image and movement sequences together that revealed a nuanced understanding of the conflictual sensations akin to the entrapment, struggle and hope experienced during phases of recovery from addiction. Indeed, the process of relation with other bodies with similar embodied experiences meant that the resonances of the felt experience of recovery emerged through the piece. Inadvertently, biographical material infused the performance, although it was morphed into symbolic references or slightly altered narratives. The following reflective comment illustrates the shared bodily knowledge that would resonate during the creative process and, I suggest, emerged into a constellation that became the performance:

SARAH: It's not about your core addiction, your prime physical addiction, it's what that creates and, even when that's taken away, it's what you were either trying to treat or fix with that. And you're left with something – and the messiness of that ... that never leaves you ... So, how do you begin to create an existence for yourself with that and where does that take your life story?

(Day one of *The Antidote* workshops)

Much of the discussion about the development of characters by each collaborator for the performance coincided with reflections on identity and the perception of being different to what one collaborator referred to as the 'norm'. They shared experiences of being marginalised, but also feelings of solidarity in identifying with a recovery identity. For instance, Sean stated,

We're also unique in a way because not everybody tackles their emotions and we have to – at your early stages [of recovery] ... Y'know, you run away and hide your emotions, but what's unique is we had to put ourselves through that, question your emotions and don't be afraid of the answer.

(Day three of *The Antidote* workshops)

I consider that this revealed the collaborators' awareness of their identity in contrast to the hegemonic value systems of the society around them. There were many moments of reflection that revealed their sense of exclusion from, or frustration with, societal notions of addiction and recovery or the systemic structures of society that reinforce marginalisation. From these comments, I infer that they were particularly aware of their own attunement but also their antagonistic relationship with society. I will return to thoughts on antagonism later in this chapter.

Tuning in with the Feeling of Sound

Given that constellations, as discussed in this chapter, incorporate nonhuman features, a discussion of tuning in with the nonhuman elements of performance seems pertinent. In FK Alexander's performance of *Recovery*, objects performed as co-actors through their production of a 'sonic milieu' (Gallagher 2016, 44) which generated the narrative content of the piece. They demonstrated the potential for 'posthumanist performativity' (Barad 2008, 121) in theatrical intra-activity between the human performer and sound-emitting objects. In particular, communication through sound rather than words revealed the potential of object-focused performance to convey aspects of experience that might otherwise by 'unspeakable' (Bernstein 2009, 70). In the context of performing experiences related to addiction and recovery, *Recovery* demonstrated that language need not be used to portray aspects of the embodied sensations of these lived experiences. Instead, the resonating objects moved the human audience to tune in with the vibrational narrative emanating from them.

I attended *Recovery* with a fellow performance researcher with whom I recorded a post-show reflection immediately after the show.[1] Two weeks later, I also recorded a reflective conversation with FK Alexander about the performance. The analysis that follows utilises observations made during both recorded conversations, as well as my memories of my own embodied experience of the performance in an attempt to convey through written language the affective experience of the performance.

FK Alexander is a performance artist 'whose work is concerned with issues of wounds, recovery, aggressive healing, radical wellness, industrialisation and noise music'.[2] As the performance began, Alexander stood in the centre of the space, bedecked in glittery costume. The spangled make-up, tousled hair and shiny bindi seemed reminiscent of the forms of attire worn by performers and clubbers at electronic dance festivals or gigs. The conflation of signifiers from the contexts of the western dance club and the theatre, while also utilising objects associated with eastern practices of transcendental meditation, was simultaneously familiar yet strange. This sensation of out-of-jointness (Thrift 2008, 14) evoked a particular bodily engagement that was paradoxically both uncomfortable and comfortable. As the objects began their performance, beginning with the hypnotic ringing of the Tibetan singing bowls which were then joined by the deep tremor of noise from the speaker stacks, these oxymoronic sensations intensified.

FK Alexander's *Recovery* was a performance communicated mainly without words, except for her introductory instructions to the audience. This was a piece that utilised affect in an innovative way in that the sight, sound, and indeed vibration, of sound-emitting objects generated a deep bodily experience. Interdisciplinary researcher Michael Gallagher defined 'sonic affect' as 'the vibrational movement of bodies of all kinds' to decentre anthropocentric notions of sound (2016, 42). He defused overemphasis on the materiality of objects and bodies, by focusing on sound as waves of movement *through* and *between* bodies which, consequently, accrue other layers of movement, such as motor responses, feelings, perceptions and memories (43). His discussion usefully equates affect as a force that is not bodily located, but moves through bodies, objects and space. This correlation of sound with movement is useful in that it relates to Manning's discussion of *being* as a series of tendencies or inclinations of movement (2013, 16). Sound waves might, therefore, be conceived as entities that exist beyond a 'body' in the quotidian sense of the word.

In *Recovery*, the 'vibrant materiality' (Bennett 2010, 13) of the sound-emitting objects operated through their power of sonic vibration that transmitted a force that moved through, and was felt by, the bodies of the audience members lying on the floor in the theatre space. Both my companion, Amy,[3] and I shared in our reflection afterwards that the sonic sensations evoked for us memories and associations with the affective experience of the process of recovery, either from addiction, illness or some other difficulty. The Tibetan singing bowls, joined by the sounds played by the 'noise DJs' over the electronic sound system, generated a milieu of sound that provoked a strong relation to the piece as a felt sensation that correlated with our own embodied understanding of what a journey of recovery might feel like. These incorporated sensations of discomfort similar to anxiety, or nausea, a dull ache in our ears and, at one point, the feeling of excess reminiscent of the sensory overload one might feel at the end of a long night of clubbing.

It was apparent from our reflections that the sounds generated by the objects, a combination of solid instruments and electronic devices, resonated in our bodies provoking an affective response. We both felt a spectrum of contradictory sensations. At first, the relaxing sound of the Tibetan singing bowls evoked memories of meditative practices, such as yoga and mindfulness activities. However, the heavier sounds from the electronic sound system felt intrusive and unsettling. Indeed, at points, the resonance was physically uncomfortable and even painful, causing our ears to ache. Presumably, this is why ear plugs were offered to us on entry to the performance. In this way, objects were indeed actants emanating a palpable 'thing-power' (Bennett 2010, 6). There was, to some extent, human intentionality behind how the objects were deployed in the performance space. It was apparent that FK Alexander had carefully choreographed layers of sound and a juxtaposition of signifiers, including sound effects such as an alarm clock, to create a provocation about recovery. For instance, her choice of costume, the use of the digital image of micro-biotic movement, how she welcomed us into the space and the leaflet given to us before entering, framed the piece within a discourse around recovery. Amy reflected that she found it difficult to relax because 'the experience was already too complex' to engage with just 'one particular set of signifiers'. In her opinion, FK Alexander had set up multiple layers within the piece, one of recovery, one of addiction and one of a 'postcolonial' critique of how eastern practices are co-opted by western recovery programmes. Gallagher's discussion of making meaning from sound, however, noted that any interpretation of sonic affect is contingent on the bodies it involves and their phenomenological response (2016, 44). Any intentionality in the performance of *Recovery* might, therefore, be considered relative to the myriad of indeterminate encounters occurring as the sound moved through different bodies, with differing embodied knowledges, sensorial responses and hearing capabilities.

According to Gallagher, it is possible to identify 'sonic tendencies' (2016, 45) that certain bodies may experience in common within certain contexts, such as dancing to music in a night club. From my reflective conversation with Amy it was clear that we did share similar bodily responses to the performance. In particular, the combination of sensations of discomfort and relaxation were, for us, a poignant reminder of the conflictual experience of recovery. As I will elaborate on later, people in recovery have an awareness of their own antagonistic relationship with their surrounding milieu. Recovery is an ongoing process of resisting relapse and moving beyond the stigmatising bounds of an 'addict' identity. Practices of recovery support the navigation of these conflicts and they assist in the effort to resolve the problems that are encountered in their milieu in so far as it enables continued progress, though always incomplete. Amy's comment below highlights how FK Alexander's *Recovery* represented this struggle, in that she felt that the convergence of the signifiers of addiction and recovery within the performance were encouraging her to develop an 'ambivalence' to addiction.

> I thought it was probably one of the closest representations to recovery that I'd experienced in performance form, which is that there were all the signifiers there of addiction, in the costume, in the whole set up of the experience … in the noise, the referencing of clubs etc., the presence of all of those things in different forms and then the suggestion that you can exist in that space without engaging in those things.
> (Personal conversation with the author in 2017)

During our conversation, she elaborated by reflecting on how recovery is an uncomfortable feeling and an internal struggle. For her, the positive impact of the performance was that it demonstrated that it is still possible to resist and become 'ambivalent' to addiction. In the performance, this is demonstrated in the persistence of the sounds of recovery, the Tibetan singing bowls throughout the performance, as well as our own persistence to continue a meditative journey.

Yaron Shyldkrot has explored in his performance research the ways in which atmospheric affects might be generated through deliberately constructed scenographic or dramaturgical arrangements (2018, 153). Using 'a constellation or assemblage of natural and aesthetic elements in a particular time', he argued that this theatrically crafted atmosphere generates an encounter that impacts upon what the participant might feel or perceive (149). Similarly, I suggest that FK Alexander had carefully composed a sonic atmosphere through her intra-actions with musical objects generating the encounter that Amy and I experienced.

In keeping with my discussion of performance in this chapter as a material constellation, I am suggesting that *Recovery* demonstrates that objects might be used to create what Gallagher referred to as a 'sonic milieu' (2016, 44). The milieu created during the performance of *Recovery* evoked, at least for me and Amy, an assemblage of the sensorial dimension of lived experiences of addiction and recovery. Without using language, the affective sensation of sound invoked feelings, memory and perceptions of sociocultural surroundings. Although our encounter with the performance was contingent upon our own embodied knowledges that impacted our perception of it, I suggest that sound and image constellated together to generate a liminal milieu in which each audience member might engage in their own subjective, affective experience. By entitling the piece *Recovery*, we were invited to engage with this theme which simultaneously implied that, according to FK Alexander, 'we are all in recovery from something' (personal conversation with the author in 2017).

Antagonism

The performance of *The Antidote* also directly addressed the experience of recovery in hostile circumstances and amid a prohibitionist environment that criminalises those with dependencies on illicit substances or, as Ettorre argued, that renders those affected by addiction as 'embodied deviants' for failing to conform to normative ideas of social acceptability (2015, 6). During the opening of *The Antidote*, the characters exhibit fear and suspicion towards each other as they endeavour to determine why they are incarcerated together. They gradually discover that what they have in common is that they are all in recovery from addiction. Forced to inhabit this confined space together, the characters demonstrate the struggle to maintain the balance of mindful relation with others as they clash with, or withdraw from, each other. As the characters begin to connect and moderate their interaction to reveal the reflexive efforts of recovery, they reach a respectful truce. Yet the play concludes abruptly and with uncertainty as they are summoned to meet an unidentified 'committee'. Recovery, within the context of this play, is depicted as a collective effort of survival amid and despite antagonism as the performers navigate the painful and the unjust as inevitable features of life.

Manning's discussion of milieu highlighted that relation with others is inherently antagonistic in that it provokes us to acknowledge difference (2007, 108). During the collaborative theatre-making process of *The Antidote*, antagonism was embraced as a natural aspect of the ecology of creative activity and also recovery practices. As I discuss this relationship with antagonism below, I propose that our approach to addressing conflict could be conceived as a form of *agonism*. A space of potentiality might, consequently, operate as a site of 'agonistic democracy' (Mouffe 2013, 7).

Mouffe's concept of radical democracy, or agonism, insisted that conflict should not be eradicated, but that confrontation should be engaged within 'common allegiance to the democratic principles of liberty and equality for all' (2013, 7). With this in mind, I do not propose recovery-engaged work as an ideal process of consensus or transformation. Instead, I suggest that commitment to a common frame of relation through a shared understanding of recovery practices that acknowledge difference and encourage reflexivity and accountability to the self and others is a form of localised agonistic politics. The liminal milieu generated during performance activity with people committed to the processes of relation encouraged by recovery practices has the potential to operate as a 'conflictual consensus' in the manner proposed by Mouffe in that antagonism might be modified into moments of collective agreement through pluralist representation and negotiation (9).

Recovery-Infused Democracy

Antagonism was palpably present during the creative process of *The Antidote*. There were several challenging moments, instances of disagreement, chaos and uncertainty. An emphasis on improvisation and self-generated characterisation, while encouraging openness to chance, led to some particularly awkward and uncomfortable moments. For instance, one member of the group began to explore how their character might exhibit misogynistic and homophobic behaviour. This led to what Mary Ann Hunter has described as a 'messy negotiation' (2008, 8) as the group collectively discussed the contribution. Care was shown in how the contribution was acknowledged as the sharing of a creative idea; however, disapproval was expressed in a candid and considered manner. In this instance, the shared commitment to recovery-orientated reflexive practices provided a mechanism for working through conflict and tension.

Group check-in routines were particularly useful in facilitating the expression of uncomfortable sensations, which were received attentively by the group and mirrored in their responses to each other. For instance, there were conflictual responses to the introduction of the written script I had drafted from the improvised material to assist with the dramaturgy of the performance. Individual perspectives were expressed during a check-in that enabled those for whom a script posed a difficulty to express the feelings of anxiety this caused. One member of the group, a trained hypnotherapist, offered a free hypnotherapy session during the break to alleviate collaborators' anxiety and another group member expressed that they preferred to have a script as a framework, but stated that 'we don't have to stick to it – there's flexibility'. Ultimately this process drew upon recovery practices that encourage honesty and reflexivity about uncomfortable sensations. Agreement was not presumed or necessary. Differing perspectives were acknowledged and could co-exist within the group.

I have found that navigating emotive responses that might include anger, fear and shame, as well as joy, are a potential feature of the milieu of working with people in recovery. While this particular group did not experience moments of extreme conflict, I have worked in circumstances where heightened friction has emerged. Addiction involves extremes of thinking, feeling and doing. Those attuned to a recovery-orientated way of life acquire the skills needed to maintain a more balanced and resilient response to engaging with the world around them. Nonetheless, under significant pressure, relapse to extreme experiences of sensation can emerge in the form of highly emotive expressions, particularly those associated with anger and shame. Indeed, the first section of *The Antidote* engaged directly with the emergence of former habits of thought, feeling and behaviour under challenging circumstances. Each character portrayed what they would consider as their addiction-orientated trait, such as controlling behaviour, aggressiveness, avoidance or denial.

A practice of reflexivity that is simultaneously supportive, respectful and challenging is crucial. I also suggest that adopting this manner of reflexivity in a theatre-making experience requires the practitioner to also embrace, and possibly even model, such reflexive practices. During *The Antidote* project, both the devising process and the performance revealed patterns of relation that indicated a recovery-engaged attunement that acknowledged difference and conflict as intrinsic to any group interaction. There was a willingness to express and engage with disagreement, and, importantly, to listen and reflect. I consider such aspects of reflexivity as heightened by the concomitant practices of recovery that were embedded in modes of peer support and accountability. These processes also resonated in the performance in how the characters of *The Antidote* revealed patterns of self-reflexivity, accountability and peer support to demonstrate the features of a recovery-engaged way of being. As discussed earlier, enhancing one's capacity for 'becoming well' involves acquiring strategies for navigating conflict and painful sensations. During the devising process and the performance itself, the group supported each other in reflecting on their collective positionality as 'in recovery' while acknowledging their differing identities within, and outside of, recovery communities.

With regard to the wider society, such performance practice has agonistic potential in its form of political representation. The processes of affective attunement in the group generated a constellation that revealed modes of communicating with others that shared knowledge of recovery from addiction. *The Antidote* performance emphasised recovery, rather than addiction. It revealed the counter-narratives of representations of people in recovery different to predominant notions of the 'addict' identity. In so doing, I consider it to perform a certain kind of agonistic activism which highlights the nuance of the lived experience of addiction and recovery and invites the audience to challenge what they think they know about the surrounding environment in which we are potentially complicit to systems of addiction.

Yet it is also important to maintain an understanding of the spatial dimension of this practice, that bodies-in-process are attuned within a facilitated space of theatrical activity. As Massey contended, spatiality is integral to any formation of political subjectivity (2005, 10). By this, she critiqued Mouffe's earlier writing on identity politics to highlight her omission of the fundamental influence of how the embedded practices that constitute any given space also inform the political identities that operate within this context (10). The practice of agonism I propose here requires more than a recognition and expression of difference, but an understanding of how difference itself is constructed by the systems of power that generate hegemonic values. The space of potentiality that I offer in performance practice might, thus, be conceived as a site of agonistic practice formed through the event of performance-making which facilitates recovery-engaged modes of relation that understand collectivity, and certainly recovery, as an ongoing negotiation.

Revealing the Obscured

Mouffe's concept of radical democracy proposes that any model of politics that founds its claims of democracy on its capacity for establishing consensus is undermined by the fallacy that a 'universal consensus' can be achieved (2013, 3). It is very evident that the contemporary political climate is composed of divergent opinions for which no resolution can be found that appeases all factions, be that Brexit, immigration or any other socio-economic policy. This simple observation confirms Mouffe's assertion that the search for universal harmony and agreement must be abandoned as an emancipatory ideal in democratic politics (2013, xi). She advocated a system of politics that embraced a 'conflictual consensus', whereby disagreeing factions might still work together under common principles (7). Disagreement is not erased; instead, conflict is converted into productive activity through pluralist representation, or what she refers to as agonism.

As shown earlier, a recovery-engaged approach to collaboration in performance-making can operate as a process of agonism through systems of negotiation and reflexivity that are accountable for the ways in which we may affect, and be affected by, others. Here, I examine how the public sharing of performances generated from bodily knowledges of addiction and insights from practices of recovery can potentially contribute to an agonistic model of society. Mouffe asserted that artistic practice can contribute to agonistic democracy by 'making visible' what the current hegemonic consensus tends to 'obscure and obliterate' (93). The assumption that 'making visible' is sufficient has been troubled by Tony Fisher's philosophical examination of 'performing agonism' (2017, 7). He argued that the political power of such performances is not what they state at the level of 'discursive statements', but 'what they show regarding the structures that produce those statements' (7). My discussion below identifies how the nonhuman elements of FK Alexander's *Recovery* reveal the antagonistic interrelations that occur between the human, nonhuman and societal systems in which experiences of addiction and recovery are enveloped. By revealing these *messy connections* the sonic performance evokes an 'aesthetics of critical visibility' (20) in how it provokes a bodily dissonance through its affective capabilities, and prompts those experiencing it to view societal values, habits and priorities from a different, felt perspective.

FK Alexander's *Recovery* particularly engages the audience in critical awareness of the conflictual features of the macro-political systems of society, specifically a postcolonial reading of western appropriation of eastern spiritual practices. As described above, FK Alexander used a variety of Tibetan singing bowls as well as a large gong in her performance. These were used to create a continuous undertone of sound throughout the performance, reminiscent of the background music used in some transcendental meditation practices. While her costume was mainly indicative of club apparel, her forehead was adorned with an exaggerated, jewelled bindi. This was, I suggest, a very deliberate choice, given criticisms at that time of appropriated use of ethnic apparel at festivals.[4]

These signifiers were performed simultaneously with electronic music and an array of sound effects indicating a habitual western lifestyle, such as the ringing of an alarm clock and church bells. During our reflective conversation after experiencing the performance, Amy commented that she felt drawn to a critical awareness of how 'we use non-western forms as a means of recovery from our own capitalist experience, our neoliberal experience'. She also indicated that it provoked her to reflect upon 'the western' as the source of addiction. FK Alexander corroborated this response during our conversation two weeks later, stating that

> capitalism has co-opted a lot of self-help, [a lot] of eastern practice or meditation and mindfulness and yoga and all these things. It's co-opted these things and turned it into this bland *Psychologies* magazine, yoga pant-wearing bullshit. And it doesn't acknowledge days when you just want to take a hammer to something.
> (Personal conversation with the author in 2017)

FK Alexander was not suggesting that meditative practices should not be used by people in recovery, rather that the commodification of these practices removes them from their original context and imposes a 'bland' westernised version that can be sold in the expanding market of the contemporary self-help 'lifestyle' industry. Of course, she is not the first to criticise the distortion of meditative practices in the west. Addiction research by Shonin et al. (2016) argued that the increasing use of a secularised version of 'mindfulness' correlates with an increasing development of addiction to 'self' or 'self-improvement'. By removing the practice of 'mindfulness' away from its original principles, mainly derived from a Buddhist spiritual practice, it becomes isolated from its original ethos of selflessness and is distorted into an obsession with the self. Sahanika Ratnayake warned, however, that the 'watering-down' and 'distortion' of these ideas in commodified versions of mindfulness 'over-simplifies the difficult business of understanding oneself' (2019). An emphasis on stepping back from one's emotions encourages a lack of critical engagement, which is not in keeping with ancient Buddhist practice and the critical reflection that is required for deep personal development that supports wellbeing.

Mindfulness and meditation can be a useful strategy for people in recovery. Although, as noted by FK Alexander in conversation with me, these practices are only one aspect of a holistic engagement in spiritual and psychological healing. For FK Alexander, meditation enables her to 'listen' and, therefore, to connect better with her 'higher power' and the world around her. Her performance of *Recovery* invites us to critically evaluate the strategies we adopt to support our wellbeing and how we use them with awareness and appreciation or, problematically, appropriate them. Returning to the political references of *Recovery*, FK Alexander's work infers that rather than address the systemic causes of addictive behaviours, we are sold sanitised versions of practices with inherently flawed promises of a good life. This resonates with Berlant's concept of cruel optimism (2010, 94) in that wellbeing is commercialised as an individually achievable package that obscures the everyday realities that are negatively impacted by systemic factors that are beyond the comprehension of the individual.

An appreciation of agonism is also evident in FK Alexander's approach to compassion. She acknowledges that she often encounters 'uncomfortable and challenging behaviour' that she attributes as the 'manifestation of the deep overwhelm of discomfort at being alive' (personal conversation with the author in 2017). In her view, all behaviour is influenced by someone's experience of relation with the world and, therefore, in her practice of recovery she considers everyone deserving of compassion. This is not a compassion that should be conflated with empathy or sympathy, but simply an acceptance of our shared experiences of vulnerability within the broader system of the 'universe'.[5] Adelina Ong's concept of compassionate mobilities is useful here in interpreting compassion as 'thoughtfulness and care that attends to the implications of an interconnected world' (2018, 10–11). Ong suggested a way forward through acceptance of difference, of conflicting 'hopes', and an appreciation of how our actions might impact on others which generates an openness towards negotiating a way of moving forward compassionately (10–11).

In FK Alexander's *Recovery*, 'self-help' commodities circulate in an affective economy in which positive value is attributed to the individual that is deemed to conform to the image of the calm, emotionally peaceful and positive expression of a citizen that takes appropriate care of their wellbeing. Alexander argued that there is a sanitising of emotion, and of politics, that inhibits recovery. In particular, she stated that 'anger is just as much an energy as anything else and lots of addicts have a lot of anger, a huge amount of anger' (personal conversation with the author). Her use of 'noise'[6] music provokes us to acknowledge the *uncomfortable* sensations of being in the world as much as the pleasurable. In his discussion of the politics of the genre of noise music, Paul Hegarty theorised the 'masochistic' effect of such performances (2013, 137). Rather than pain or eroticism, he applied the Deleuzian concept of masochism as 'not about suffering but about dis-organising and reorganising the world through physical activity' (138) to the experience of a noise performance. Drawing on his reading of this music genre, I suggest that FK Alexander's use of noise in *Recovery* served to unsettle the audience from a comfortable, uncritical position by reorientating our perspective through the sonic affects of the piece.

Conclusion

In summary, both *The Antidote* and *Recovery* generated liminal milieus infused by bodily experiences of practices of recovery. In the case of *The Antidote*, by forming a temporary environment through collaborative theatre-making informed by past experiences and contemporary sociopolitical context, but not bound by them, we were able to reimagine how to share a certain way of being in the world. We demonstrated our commitment and capacity to affect and be affected through and beyond the theatrical experience. In sharing the resultant constellation as a public performance, we showed that people in recovery might contribute to a more pluralist representation of society through the sharing of perspectives that are often hidden or obscured.

Alternatively, the nonhuman performers in Alexander's *Recovery* created a sonic atmosphere, reminding us of the nonhuman, or more-than-human, dimension of addiction and recovery. Their sonic affects intermittently soothe and jar us into a critical visibility of how human-centred society inhibits capacities for 'becoming well' (Duff 2016). Both examples illustrate the productive ways in which artistic practice can generate atmospheres of recovery.

Notes

1 The post-show conversation with a colleague assisted in translating the traces of the affective sensation of the performance felt through our bodies to a linguistic form of expression for the purpose of analysing the experience for my research. While this might have resulted in us applying our own cultural and disciplinary references to the experience, thus altering it, it was useful to compare our reflections with the subsequent conversation I had with FK Alexander to discover whether her artistic intentions had been received and understood by us through the performance.
2 https://www.artsadmin.co.uk/profiles/fk-alexander/.
3 Name changed to protect anonymity.
4 During the summers of 2017 and 2018, there was a particular emphasis in online magazines and news media on raising awareness of cultural appropriation in festival attire and encouraging festival-goers to avoid wearing outfits that might cause offence to ethnic minorities. See, for example, https://www.buzzfeed.com/sohanjudge/cultural-appropriation-festival-fashion (accessed 17 September 2018).

5 The term 'universe' is often used in recovery circles to refer to a 'higher power' that is not necessarily a deity, but rather a recognition that humans are part of a bigger ecology of systems of life beyond our control. It is often adopted by people who do not practice a particular religion, but need to develop their understanding of spirituality if they are following the Twelve Steps programme of recovery (Ducoat 2018).
6 Noise is a genre of avant-garde music considered to have emerged in 1980s and, according to Hegarty, has a close association with 'very physical performance art' (2013, 135). As an art form, it resists structure and the usual sonic conventions of music and so is associated with transgressive politics (133–134).

References

Ahmed, S. (2014) *The cultural politics of emotion*. 2nd ed. Edinburgh: Edinburgh University Press.

Barad, K. (2008) 'Posthumanist performativity: Towards an understanding of how matter comes to matter', in S. Alaimo and S. Hekman (eds), *Material feminisms*. Bloomington: Indiana University Press, pp. 120–154.

Bennett, J. (2010) *Vibrant matter: A political ecology of things*. Durham, NC: Duke University Press.

Berlant, L. (2010) 'Cruel optimism', in M. Gregg and G.J. Seigworth (eds), *The affect theory reader*. Durham, NC: Duke University Press, pp. 94–117.

Bernstein, R. (2009) 'Dances with things', *Social Text*, 27 (4), pp. 67–94. Available at: https://doi.org/10.1215/01642472-2009-055.

Brown, C.B. (2012) *Daring greatly: How the courage to be vulnerable transforms the way we live, love, parent, and lead*. 1st ed. New York: Gotham Books.

Ducoat, I. (2018) 'A Higher Power for those who don't believe in a Higher Power', *Psychcentral*, 7 August. Available at: https://psychcentral.com/blog/a-higher-power-for-those-who-dont-believe-in-a-higher-power/ (accessed 12 August 2019).

Duff, C. (2016) 'Atmospheres of recovery: Assemblages of health', *Environment and Planning A*, 48 (1), pp. 58–74. Available at: https://doi.org/10.1177/0308518X15603222.

Ettorre, E. (2015) 'Embodied deviance, gender, and epistemologies of ignorance: Revisioning drugs use in a neurochemical, unjust world', *Substance Use & Misuse*, 50 (6), pp. 794–805. Available at: https://doi.org/10.3109/10826084.2015.978649.

Fisher, T. (2017) 'Introduction: Performance and the tragic politics of the Agōn', in T. Fisher and E. Katsouraki (eds), *Performing antagonism: Theatre, performance and radical democracy*. London: Palgrave Macmillan, pp. 1–20.

Gallagher, M. (2016) 'Sound as affect: Difference, power and spatiality', *Emotion, Space and Society*, 20, pp. 42–48. Available at: https://doi.org/10.1016/j.emospa.2016.02.004.

Hegarty, P. (2013) 'Brace and embrace: Masochism in noise performance', in M. Thompson and I. Biddle (eds), *Sound, music, affect: Theorising sonic experience*. London and New York: Bloomsbury, pp. 133–146.

Hunter, M.A. (2008) 'Cultivating the art of safe space', *Research in Drama Education: The Journal of Applied Theatre and Performance*, 13 (1), pp. 5–21. Available at: https://doi.org/10.1080/13569780701825195.

Manning, E. (2007) *Politics of touch: Sense, movement, sovereignty*. Minneapolis: University of Minnesota Press.

Manning, E. (2013) *Always more than one: Individuation's dance*. Durham, NC: Duke University Press.

Massey, D.B. (2005) *For space*. London and Thousand Oaks, CA: SAGE.

Mouffe, C. (2013) *Agonistics: Thinking the world politically*. London and New York: Verso.

Nicholson, H. (2014) *Applied drama: The gift of theatre*. 2nd ed. Basingstoke and New York: Palgrave Macmillan.

Ong, A. (2018) 'The limits of access: The messy temporalities of hope and the negotiation of place', *Research in Drama Education: The Journal of Applied Theatre and Performance*, 23 (3), pp. 467–478. Available at: https://doi.org/10.1080/13569783.2018.1468242.

Ratnayake, S. (2019) 'The problem of mindfulness', *Aeon*, 25 July. Available at: https://aeon.co/essays/mindfulness-is-loaded-with-troubling-metaphysical-assumptions.

Sedgwick, E.K. and Frank, A. (2003) *Touching feeling: Affect, pedagogy, performativity*. Durham, NC: Duke University Press.

Shonin, E., Van Gordon, W. and Griffiths, M.D. (2016) 'Ontological addiction: Classification, etiology, and treatment', *Mindfulness*, 7 (3), pp. 660–671. Available at: https://doi.org/10.1007/s12671-016-0501-4.

Shyldkrot, Y. (2018) 'Mist opportunities: Haze and the composition of atmosphere', *Studies in Theatre and Performance*, pp. 1–18. Available at: https://doi.org/10.1080/14682761.2018.1505808.

Thompson, J. (2011) *Performance affects: Applied theatre and the end of effect*. Basingstoke and New York: Palgrave Macmillan.

Thrift, N.J. (2008) *Non-representational theory: Space, politics, affect*. Abingdon and New York: Routledge.

Zontou, Z. (2017) 'Upon awakening: Addiction, performance, and aesthetics of authenticity', in A. O'Grady (ed.), *Risk, participation, and performance practice: Critical vulnerabilities in a precarious world*. New York: Palgrave Macmillan, pp. 205–231.

3 Objects of Addiction and Recovery in Artistic Practice

During the summer of October 2016, I watched a performance of Headlong Theatre's production of Duncan Macmillan's *People, Places, Things* at Wyndham's Theatre in London. The title of the play highlighted what has been discussed already throughout this book, that the experience of addiction is propelled by a person's surroundings. Anna Harpin's analysis of the play noted that Macmillan engages with the 'corrosive impact of capitalism on belonging, connection and human worth' (2018, 161). Emma,[1] the play's protagonist, emphasised the influence of contextual environment on recovery in a speech made to the audience.

> They tell you, in rehab they tell you: avoid people who make you want to relapse. Places you associate with using and objects that might be a trigger. People, places and things. That's basically, you know, *everything*. As long as you steer clear of people, places and things you'll be fine.
>
> (Macmillan 2015, 129)

Many addiction treatment programmes consider past associations in human and nonhuman form as potential triggers for relapse. Yet, as Macmillan's character states, 'That's basically, you know, *everything*'. It is these past connections that form the materiality of a person's lived experience during recovery. While it may be possible, and advisable, to avoid potential triggers of relapse, adopting a life of recovery is much more complex than simply avoiding certain influences. For instance, past associations also involve the histories, family relations, socio-economic conditions, sociopolitical structures, media representations and societal attitudes that impact upon a person's experience of, and relation to, the world around them and, therefore, their recovery process in it. Applying Duff's assemblage approach to understanding addiction develops an awareness of the complex and multiple factors impacting on a person's emergent capacity for 'becoming well' (2016, 58). An emphasis on the societal factors that contribute to psychological crisis has also been emphasised in Harpin's *Beyond Illness: Madness, Art and Society*. For instance, she proposed that we resist pathologising Macmillan's Emma and, instead, consider

DOI: 10.4324/9781003271062-4

her addiction as a 'coping mechanism' for pain and distress intensified by sociopolitical context (2018, 140).

To extend my discussion of recovery-engaged performance practice as an affective ecology, it is useful to further investigate the connections such performances have with the sociopolitical world that surrounds them. To understand fully how performance practice can operate in a recovery-engaged way, I examine the manner in which identities of recovery, and indeed the pejorative label of 'addict', are informed by their societal context. Consequently, in this chapter, I extend my discussion of the concept of milieu, discussed in Chapters 1 and 2, to explore the material, nonhuman aspect of recovery-engaged arts practices. Specifically, in this chapter I observe how objects perform to assist in the telling of stories of addiction and recovery. The discussion draws on two different examples of practice created with and by people with experience of recovery from addiction. The first is Simon Mason's performance of *Too High Too Far Too Soon*, during which objects operated as dramaturgical tools. The second is Portraits of Recovery's (PORe) participatory art project staged in Manchester in 2022, the Repair Centre, which harnessed the Japanese art of Kintsugi, a philosophy through which the repair of a broken object is left visible rather than concealed (Kemske 2021). I focus on objects in this chapter to demonstrate how they contribute to revealing the 'assemblages' of addiction that posthumanist addiction research considered vital for developing a better understanding of the contextualised experience of addiction (Duff 2014; Dennis and Farrugia 2017). The nonhuman performances in arts practices by or with people in recovery have, as yet, been unexplored.

My attention to the affective force of material things builds upon concepts of material agency proposed, specifically, by Bennett (2010) and Barad (2008). Barad's discussion of 'posthumanist performativity' is useful to my discussion of artistic practice in that it refutes the division of the human and nonhuman as separate entities and, instead, suggests that both have agency through their 'intra-actions' with each other (2008, 144). Bennett's vital materialism also affords agency to the nonhuman and her discussion of this as a form of ethics is useful to my discussion in this chapter that reinforces my exploration of objects in performance as potentially supporting the ethical and political imperatives of recovery-engaged performance practice. By attributing agency to objects through her concept of 'thing-power', Bennett challenged us to consider the world around us as an interconnected web in which all things are considered vital contributors (2010, 12–13). It is perhaps obvious how Bennett's vital materialism is useful in the field of environmentalism to reconsider how we privilege human desire for consumption over the harm caused to the very elements of the nonhuman environment that we depend upon for survival. In this chapter, however, I suggest that vital materialism assists in challenging systemic assumptions and approaches towards recovery from addiction through revealing how societal contexts generate *affects* – and assemblages (Duff 2014, 132) – that compound addiction and hinder recovery. As a performance researcher, I am interested in what emerges from analysing socially engaged performance as a vital materiality. How might performers, objects, theatrical space and place resonate to create a constellation of the material features of lived experiences of addiction and recovery? Specifically, how might performances generated from a recovery-engaged ethos, including lived experience of addiction, offer a distinctly affective portrayal of interaction with objects, or the nonhuman, that reveal the material realities of addiction and recovery? How might this generate new ways of knowing, thinking and intra-acting about recovery, as well as about performance practice?

The Vibrancy of 'Objects of Addiction' as Dramaturgical Tools

Too High Too Far Too Soon was a collaboration between Simon Mason and Outside Edge Theatre during which I worked with Mason to devise and stage his published autobiography (Mason 2013).[2] The lived experience shared in this autobiography entailed a struggle with addiction spanning more than 20 years of his life as well as, at one point, involvement in the supply of recreational substances to many Britpop celebrities. The stage version of *Too High Too Far Too Soon* was performed by him at the Tristan Bates Theatre in London from 25 November to 20 December 2014, having toured a number of addiction treatment centres across England in early November. It was subsequently performed in individual showings at venues in Liverpool, Manchester and London in 2015. For the purpose of developing my discussion of the performative potential of intra-action with inorganic material in this chapter, I critically reflect on how objects, specifically those that might be referred to as 'props', performed as 'vibrant' dramaturgical devices in the making and performance of *Too High Too Far Too Soon*. In developing my consideration of the ethical and political dimensions of recovery-engaged performance practice, I adapt Ahmed's concept of 'sticky affect' (2010, 29) to offer an approach to working with objects that accounts for the affects they may evoke for people in recovery, particularly their potential to trigger cravings or painful memories. In my discussion of Mason's use of objects related to addiction in *Too High Too Far Too Soon*, I suggest that the material features of the performance can not only illustrate more accurately the contextualised experience of addiction but can also disrupt pejorative stereotypes as well as enabling the performer (and possibly the spectator) to renegotiate their previous intra-action with these 'things' by engaging with them differently during the theatrical encounter.

Too High Too Far Too Soon was an unusual project during which I worked with the verbatim narrative of someone's autobiographical story. In my prior work with Outside Edge Theatre Company, I was accustomed to collaborating with people in recovery to create performances inspired by issues and themes relevant to their lived experiences, but not to their actual life stories. As discussed in Chapter 2, risk and vulnerability are features of recovery-engaged practice; nonetheless, helping a performer to re-enact past experiences that may instigate a re-experiencing of trauma brings additional risk. This is all the more so if such risk-taking might trigger relapse. There is also an aesthetic risk, or what O'Grady has coined as a 'risky aesthetics' (2017, x). Zontou noted, in relation to the work of the Fallen Angels Dance Theatre company, that 'the dramatization of personal experiences of addiction contains in its core the dramatization of stigma' (2014, 343). Framed and balanced appropriately in performance, it can challenge stereotypes of addiction and politicise the reality of addiction and recovery. Alternatively, it can, as Zontou stated, 'create ambivalence through reinforcing familiar stereotypes' (348).

In the case of *Too High Too Far Too Soon*, Mason had already published his autobiography and was committed to developing it into a performance which could be shared with others in the hope that it might demonstrate the possibility of recovery to others who might connect with the narrative. The project had been set up by my predecessor at Outside Edge, Phil Fox; in stepping into his role as artistic director I took on the task of staging Mason's story. It was a project that posed particular challenges from the outset and I do not suggest that my solutions were ideal. By critically reflecting on the strategies used, however, I suggest that a 'vital materialism' (Bennett 2010, 12–13) operated that demonstrates the potential of object-focused work in recovery arts.

It became apparent in the early stages of rehearsing the performance that objects would be vital for the piece. One of the discoveries I have encountered when working with people who have a prior history of heavy substance abuse is that neurological change may have occurred that impact short-term memory and recall.[3] Mason's memory was similarly affected. On the first day of rehearsal it was evident that he was struggling with using the script that I had drafted from our development discussions. Realising that the prospect of having to memorise such a large amount of material was hindering his connection to the rehearsal process, we agreed to set aside the script and adopt a more improvised approach. After all, this was about Mason's life story and inevitably he embodied the narrative. As the director, however, I was keen to support Mason's performance by finding a way to evoke his connection to past memories as well as devising a system for dramaturgically structuring the improvised material into a coherent narrative for the audience.

My initial approach was to consider how to plot key moments of narrative from Mason's autobiography to evoke time, place and affect that would become a tangible performance of his experience. Committed to a collaborative approach to theatre-making predicated on Mason having autonomy over what was ultimately his life story, we searched for a process that Mason could use confidently in performance. Objects became an effective mechanism to achieve this. For instance, the nickname of Mason's dealer was the 'cat in the hat'. Hats became, subsequently, a useful mechanism to indicate key periods in his life. During the devising stages, I carefully negotiated with Mason which objects might assist him in reconnecting with the pieces of his life story that we had agreed to include in the theatrical performance. From this, I created a living diagram in the rehearsal space to create a topography of the narrative, thereby relating objects to place and time. As each object was positioned and moved around on stage they prompted Mason's largely improvised storytelling.

Bennett's 'thing-power' purports to 'the curious ability of inanimate things to animate, to act, to produce effects dramatic and subtle' (2010, 6). As dramaturgical devices, the props in *Too High Too Far Too Soon* demonstrated a 'thing-power' as actants that evoked the narrative from Mason. Resonating together with him in the liminal space of the rehearsal, and later, performance venue, they formed the constellation of a contextualised performance of a struggle with addiction situated in the time-space of Mason's life. In keeping with my discussion of theatre-making in Chapters 1 and 2, intra-action with these objects generated a space of potentiality. By this, it formed a liminal milieu (a non-normative expanded time-space) in which he could revisit embodied memories and review and renegotiate his relationship with these objects in the present. The convergence of past with present, including a current practice of recovery, combined with our experimentation with theatrical forms of communicating moments of his experience to an audience, instigated the potential features and affects of the resultant performance.

In 'Dances with Things', Robin Bernstein argued that objects and elements of material culture *script* human actions (2009, 68). She proposed that a 'scriptive thing' cues culturally embedded responses from the human while also allowing for resistance or variation in response (69). Of particular relevance to my reflections on *Too High Too Far Too Soon* is her discussion of how objects may become scriptive things through triggering 'kinesthetic imagination' as a 'faculty of memory' (70). Building on Joseph Roach's original use of the concept of kinesthesia in performance, she demonstrated that 'dancing with things', or thinking through movement with objects, can assist with expressing what might otherwise remain 'unspeakable' (70). In the context of *Too High Too Far Too Soon*, playing with things such as hats, photographs, vinyl records, foil, bags of powder and a brightly coloured blanket bought at a music festival enabled Mason to simultaneously remember and reinvent moments of experience through new encounters with these things as theatrical objects. As Bernstein stated, 'Things invite us to dance, and when we sweep them onto the dance floor, they appear animate' (70).

Frequently, the performance with these objects revealed their scripted tendencies within the occasions of drug culture portrayed in the piece. For instance, the chopping of white powder with a card, the rolling of foil, or the 'dealing' of sweets to the audience induced codes of bodily response from Mason that revealed the patterns of sociability within the context of the world of his autobiography. His hands, body, even breath, would respond in habitual attunement with objects indicative of drug paraphernalia. The vinyl records, and selected music tracks chosen from them, invoked the atmosphere of the particular music culture – and industry – in which Mason circulated; from the 'alternative' and 'indie' rock bands that performed at the Glastonbury festivals of the late 1980s to the Britpop artists of the 1990s. Again, Mason's body would mould itself in response to the specific timbre of the music, whether played over the speaker system or inferred by holding a record. Often, this was associated with certain substance-influenced bodily sensations, such as the giggly euphoria of acid to 'The Whole of The Moon' by The Waterboys (Ensign Records 1985) or the cocaine-induced posturing to 'Cigarettes and Alcohol' by Oasis (Creation 1994).

Conversely, we played with resistance to past attunement with such items. The 'sweets', performing the role of ecstasy tablets, were imprinted with 'Like Me'. This inscription was a suggestion from Mason to convey his realisation, in recovery, that a significant motivating factor of his behaviour as a dealer was the desire to be 'liked', to feel inclusion and belonging. I suggest that the presence of the inscription on the sweets subtly subverted, at least for Mason, their prior script as drug commodities. The incorporation of atypical objects for a 'drug assemblage' (Duff 2014, 127), such as family photographs, a child's beach bucket and a toy aeroplane, were also deployed to disrupt an easy stereotype of Mason's world. The juxtaposition of these items on stage indicated that narratives of addiction are complex, contextual and do not begin with an 'addict'. Rather, the addict identity that Mason came to inhabit emerged through years of intra-action with objects, substances and other human bodies that became the assemblage of the idiosyncratic experience of his life as a drug user, drug dealer and, latterly, a person in recovery.

I was not entirely comfortable with our reliance on objects, however, particularly because the association of several of our objects with addiction raised ethical dilemmas. Many of our selected objects were indicative of drug paraphernalia and I was mindful of the fact that they could evoke potentially powerful affective resonances. Neurobiologist Marc Lewis in *The Biology of Desire* (2016) outlined how images or items, such as a needle or a vein, can trigger neural activity connected to the brain's reward-seeking system which in turn triggers the desire for the object of addiction, be that heroin, a cigarette or 'chocolate cheesecake' (57–58). Indeed, substances, and objects related to the rituals of their use, have often been anthropomorphised in songs, poetry and performance.

My reference here to anthropomorphism does not seek to attribute human features to objects of addiction, but rather to draw attention to the emotional attachments triggered by such objects. In this regard, Ahmed's concept of 'sticky affect' is useful in that she demonstrated that objects become associated with certain emotions, such as happiness, which determines social actions by generating an orientation either towards or away from the object (2010, 29). A 'happy object', according to Ahmed, pulls a person towards it with the illusory promise of 'feeling good' to which it has become attached (29). In the context of addiction, a piece of foil, a spoon, or a particular style of music, might be 'sticky' with the affective force of promises of a 'high' or analgesic relief from other sources of pain. For someone affected by addiction these objects become happy objects, although they may transpire to be 'cruel' in the manner that Berlant suggests (2010, 95). I was concerned, therefore, that such props might trigger a relapse either for Mason or for those in recovery who viewed the performance. The process of working with these objects highlighted for me, as a practitioner, the importance of working alongside someone in understanding their own process of recovery, negotiating boundaries and having an affective attunement to Mason throughout the rehearsal and performance process. As discussed in Chapter 2, I suggest that bodily attunement occurs during the creative process through a sharing of, and tuning in to, bodily sensations and knowledges of recovery.

It is possible that I attributed too much power to the objects as a trigger for relapse. Indeed, given that the process of recovery is contingent upon the unique convergence of experiences and practices of each individual, or each body-in-process, relapse triggers can be quite subjective and also relative to the length and stability of the practice of recovery.[4] Ironically, reflecting on the performance in a reflexive conversation with him in 2016, Mason told me that it was not the scene in which he used a syringe needle, belt and spoon to simulate an attempted overdose of heroin that he found difficult, but instead a scene that was not directly related to drugs; it was the scene in which he, at the age of eleven, returns home from school to discover that his father has died. Having been abstinent from substance use for over eight years at the time of the project, he found that it was not the objects of addiction, such as foil or needles that were a potential trigger, but the *imagined* objects, such as the bed in which his father died, that were attached to powerful feelings. This highlighted to me that, in this practice, it might not be the seemingly obvious addiction-related features that might trigger intense responses that could potentially disrupt recovery.

Ahmed's concept of emotion as shaped by objects is, therefore, useful in appraising the emotive potential of objects used, and inferred, in the narrative of *Too High Too Far Too Soon*. She posited that emotions are inherently formed through our contact with objects, either material or imagined (2014, 6). Emotions are shaped by objects which are simultaneously shaped by the emotions we attach to them (7), or to use her earlier phrase, objects become 'sticky' with affect (2010, 29). This 'stickiness' binds certain values to an object, such as the promise of happiness, that increases their status as a social commodity and increases our orientation towards them (29). Within the context of Mason's life, substances, and associated paraphernalia and objects of that lifestyle, shaped his experience of the world through their value as sources of analgesia, happiness, financial gain, inclusion and acceptance. The scene that we entitled 'The Medicate Equation'[5] highlighted how Mason's orientation towards substances was inscribed by an attempt to escape sources of pain. In this scene, the eleven-year-old Mason returns home from boarding school to see his ill father, only to discover that he has died. The sequence of distress that follows culminates in Mason being given a sedative by the family GP to alleviate, although ultimately to stall, his emotional volatility. On an imaginary chalkboard, the adult Mason notes the equation he learnt that day: Feelings + Medication = No Feelings. Throughout the rest of the performance legal and illicit drugs become shaped by their value of analgesia, by the numbing of the painful sensation of the loss of a primary caregiver, and later the anesthetising of feelings associated with other traumatic events experienced in Mason's life.

The emotional value of the objects used in *Too High Too Far Too Soon* had indeterminate and contingent qualities which reveals the complexity of any ethical considerations in this type of work. For instance, with regard to the following three objects used in the 'Rockbottom – OD' scene, a needle, a teaspoon and a belt, the affective response to these objects will be influenced by the resonances of past emotion, or 'sticky affect', that are associated with them. For one person, a teaspoon might have everyday associations of tea-making or dessert-eating. For a heroin user it may be associated with 'cooking' a substance in preparation for a fix. For some people in recovery, it may not be the spoon that could act as a trigger for relapse, but a picture of a family member or a memento from childhood. The materiality of the life of someone in recovery is imbued with past associations and potential triggers. Recovery involves a daily navigation, supported by recovery practices or rituals, of encounters with people, places or things that might generate the affective lure to 'use'. Hence the adage in recovery programmes, 'just for today'.

As O'Grady's discussion of risky aesthetics emphasised, riskiness is contingent upon the specific context of practice, but it can also be purposeful for performance practice that is committed to 'openness as meaningful encounter and exchange' (2017: ix). The project of *Too High Too Far Too Soon* was premised on Mason's openness to sharing his autobiography with the intention that it might resonate with others affected by addiction. Given that *Too High Too Far Too Soon* was to be performed for audiences in addiction treatment venues, as well as to a public theatre-going audience, it is useful to distinguish how different performance settings impacted on the ethical implications of using our chosen objects in performance. Some of our performance venues included residential and community-based treatment facilities where some people might be in the early stages of detox.[6] The relative level of risk involved in performing with our chosen objects was, therefore, heightened. In early recovery, when attachment to the objects that might deliver the promise of a high are still potentially overpowering, I suggest that the lure to 'use' is too strong to risk using such items in either creative workshops or performances. In the final stages of rehearsal, we created an alternative version of the performance to omit objects that we considered too risky for use with an audience in early recovery.

During the tour of addiction treatment centres, we did not use the needle, spoon or powders. Perhaps for this audience, who already had an especially close attunement to the omitted objects, their presence was palpable enough through Mason's bodily gestures. For instance, when Mason mimed his preparation and injection of the 'hit' of heroin for the 'overdose' scene, the treatment centre audiences demonstrated attentiveness and emotive response to his actions. We were mindful that, for some, even imagined objects were 'scriptive things' (Bernstein 2009, 70). Support staff were, of course, present throughout to assist anyone who might need to leave the room and to follow up on any particular issues raised. Also, every performance within treatment settings was concluded with a post-show discussion with Mason, facilitated by me, to allow audience members to express their immediate responses, ask questions and talk about aspects of the performance or recovery. These exchanges tended to reveal a particular attunement with those in the room and Mason to the bodily and contextual dimensions of lived experience of addiction. Frequently, expressions of gratitude were shared and feelings of hope in response to Mason's sharing of his own experience.

With the permission of the addiction support staff in each treatment service venue, we used the sweets that, as mentioned earlier, Mason would deal out to the audience 'in role' as the 'cat in the hat' drug dealer. There were interesting differences in responses to the sweets from the public theatre performances compared to the treatment centre performances. Many of the audience members from the public theatre performances who received a sweet simply ate it, whereas many of those in the treatment centre context did not. We found that the sweets were either returned to us, or left on the seats. One person approached us afterwards and shared, on returning the sweet, how proud she was to resist the urge to eat it and instead hand it back. It occurred to me that perhaps we had inadvertently offered an opportunity to develop a different relation with addiction-based things. In this instance, a sweet used as a prop ecstasy pill had perhaps enabled a practice of recovery behaviour. By this I do not mean to advocate the use of drug paraphernalia in applied theatre work with people in early recovery. In reflecting on this accidental discovery, I suggest that there is potential in exploring further how objects or even place, imaginary or real, might be used within a creative, liminal space to reimagine problematic 'things' and develop an altered relation to them.

In *Too High Too Far Too Soon* the assemblage of objects on stage, accompanied by fragments of songs chosen by Mason, created a liminal milieu of the lived reality of his addiction and recovery. Rather than eroticising objects of addiction, we hoped that the discarded debris of the remnants of scattered powder, empty cans, crumpled money and so on might instead suggest the banality of these items and so pose a contrast to the power they might otherwise conjure as craved substances. In the penultimate scene, Mason swept the floor clean, replacing the detritus with a framed photo of his daughter. I would suggest that the simultaneity of past and present experience performed on stage not only supported Mason in demonstrating an altered relationship with such objects, but also indicated to those who were open to change that moving beyond addiction is possible. Our chosen objects were 'vibrant' in their contribution to the performance as dramaturgical devices that evoked from Mason a performative response. The narrative of the overall performance, therefore, emerged from the way in which Mason moved and responded to the objects. Their performance was not merely as 'scriptive things', drawing on past bodily attunement to reveal the contextualised experience of Mason's addiction, but also contributed to a space of potentiality in which new forms of relation with such items could be performed.

Objects as Narratives of Repair

While objects in theatrical performance can reveal the material assemblages of addiction, I am interested in how objects also contribute to assemblages of recovery. Indeed, how might broken or discarded objects assist in re-evaluating human-centric values regarding repair and recovery? PORe's participatory art project, the Repair Centre, provides an example in which objects were central to creative exploration of themes related to recovery from addiction.

Two days before the tea parties held to celebrate the Queen's Platinum Jubilee bank holiday weekend (2–5 June 2022), the decorative scars of the bone china teacups, saucers and plates collated for the Repair Centre were exhibited to the public at the Manchester Craft and Design Centre. These pieces of crockery unashamedly displayed their golden or multicoloured joins. The fracture-lines of two plates in particular captured my attention as I noticed the pieces of paper wedged in the gold embossed cracks, offering words of provocation such as 'needless', 'overload', 'ally' and 'fortune'. While I cannot tell what these words mean in a linguistic context, it is the gesture emerging from the site of brokenness that sticks with me.

PORe is currently the only organisation in the UK focused specifically on curating recovery-engaged art exhibits with, by and for people in recovery. The founder, Mark Prest, has been a key figure in the development of a socially engaged recoverist arts movement, coining the term in 2013 while working with Clive Parkinson, Director of Manchester Metropolitan University's arts for health unit, on an EU arts project. In conversation with him on 10 April 2018, he stated that he utilised the terms 'recoverism' and 'recoverist' as a 'means to reclaim the recovery agenda as allied to the arts'. He saw this as linking to a wider social movement that was 'softly political' in its aim to 'make visible' representations of recovery community (conversation with the author). He considered his arts practice, involving an array of socially engaged participatory art projects, as a way of 'taking back control' of the community's representation through cultural production; specifically aiming to use 'high art' to challenge the subject of recovery from addiction (conversation with the author). At the time of our initial conversation, Prest was in the process of completing a large project entitled Unseen: Simultaneous Realities which focused specifically on visibility involving careful representations of LGBTQ+ and also South Asian experiences of recovery. One of the neon signs created during this project can still be found attached to a balcony at the Rochdale train and bus interchange, proudly illuminating the haiku: 'Listen to my pulse, And walk tall I, Free like river water, Let me be.' Four years later, his most recent project shifts issues of representation further by celebrating the complex and imperfect stories of recovery.

PORe's pop-up exhibition at the Manchester Craft and Design Centre (31 May–1 June 2022) offered members of the general public the opportunity to view – and touch – artworks created by participants in the Repair Centre project. During this participatory art project, people with lived experience of recovery engaged in workshops, talks and artistic collaboration with professional artists. In the process, participants could develop specific skills, such as working with ceramics and textiles. The learning of transferable skills was, as indicated on PORe's website, one of the key aims of the project. This is unsurprising given its funding by the Greater Manchester Education and Skills Funding Agency. The Repair Centre, however, offered much more than its impact-orientated objectives claim.

As with my discussion of props in *Too High Too Far Too Soon*, the objects collated for the Repair Centre had a 'vibrant materiality', an agency in their own right, capable of evoking an affective response from the human viewer. Harris and Holman Jones in their *Queer Life of Things* remind us that objects are 'transistors' that not only preserve memories from the past but can make new impressions in the present (2019, 64). In particular, when objects challenge us to attune differently with them, they become an 'orientating force' by which we might see them as if for the very first time (65 and 66). This has powerful resonances with practices of recovery in that, as discussed in previous chapters, recovery from addiction requires a reorientation of past relations with the surrounding environment to develop less harmful ways of being. The plates used by the Repair Centre and the items of upcycled clothing and other mended objects call on us to attune differently, to see anew these objects that might have been previously discarded as imperfect or irreparable. These reimagined objects operate as transistors of lived experience of recovery, both literally in terms of their own repair and also metaphorically in relation to their encounter with the human being in addiction recovery who intra-acted with the object to create the artwork.

In conversation with Prest in 2023, he revealed to me his belief that the philosophy of Kintsugi was akin to recovery from addiction because 'it's looking at how the broken, once reconfigured and reformulated, becomes more valuable and significant than it was before'. Bonnie Kemske, one of the professional artists involved in the project, describes the ceramic art of Kinsugi as a 'poetic mend' in that it transforms a broken object into a new entity (2021, 12). Charting the historic origins of this lacquer craft in Japan from the late sixteenth to the early seventeenth centuries, Kemske highlights the cultural significance of this art as not only a practice of fixing precious items associated with loved ones but also born of a philosophy that accepts breakage and imperfection as an inherent aspect of life (14 and 17). Kemske's involvement in the Repair Centre suggests an attention to embracing the original philosophy of the art form within the project in addition to the teaching of the practical skills involved. Her metaphor of Kinstugi as a process of 'acceptance, resilience and renewal' (26) during challenging times resonates with the themes integral to practices of recovery from addiction discussed in this book.

As we emerge from the COVID-19 pandemic, there has been an increased interest in performance research on the theme of repair, such as Sue Mayo's *Breaks and Joins* participatory arts project (London, 2020–2022) and a special edition of Performance Research, *On Repair* (2021). Discussions of Kintsugi as a coping mechanism for supporting wellbeing during the pandemic have appeared in the *British Medical Journal* (Selman 2021) and the *Canadian Family Physician* (Dobkin 2022), as well as in other popular magazines. For the Northern Irish ceramicist, Rachel Ho, Kintsugi is important to her work in that it is a repair, 'but the wounds are still there and it must bear witness to the stories' (Mayo n.d.). Speaking to Sue Mayo on a podcast for the Breaks and Joins project, Ho expressed that it was important 'not just to guild over it like it never happened'. Her emphasis on witnessing and honouring stories relates closely with practices of recovery, particularly in relation to the tradition in Twelve Steps support groups of sharing stories of 'experience, strength and hope'. As with other examples of recovery-engaged performance practices throughout this book, the objects collated for the Repair Centre perform a critical visibility in that they honour the scars of the past, rather than conceal them. Moving beyond Mouffe's politics of 'revealing the obscured' (2013, 93), they invite us to appreciate, even cherish, the unconventional beauty of narratives of recovery. Might we then, in attuning differently to such narratives, begin to understand the potential of recovery-engaged arts to instigate atmospheres of recovery?

Recovery is an ongoing and collaborative process that is imperfect, sometimes painful and complex. 'Becoming well' (Duff 2016, 58) is hindered by environmental assemblages that are also broken in their perpetuity of prejudice, exploitation and harm. Peter Eckersall and Helena Grehan's editorial positions the art of repair as 'a responsibility and an ethic' that requires a sensitivity to 'brokenness' (2021, 2). While they allude to environmental, political and economic imperatives for repair, their call for a right to repair highlights practices such as survival and sustainability. Yet how does one survive a broken system? Moten and Harney's 'undercommons of fugitive study' embraces a living with brokenness (2013, 9) which is apt for my reflection on recovery-engaged arts. In particular, their emphasis on hapticality describes the undercommons as a felt entity (98). Like Moten and Harney's fugitive study, the activity of the Repair Centre facilitated tentative comings into relation with human and nonhuman in a form of messy communion with the human and nonhuman – a being together in brokenness and survival.

Reflecting on one of the ceramic workshops for the project blog,[7] creative producer Jenny Walker noted that the artistic process enabled participants to question what it means to reconstruct ourselves, but in an unconventional way. These objects, it would seem, led participants on a reflexive journey. As with *Too High Too Far Too Soon* discussed earlier, the artistic craft activities facilitated a space of potentiality in which 'dancing with things' (Bernstein 2009, 70) enabled expressions of feeling that might otherwise be untranslatable into spoken word. Elaine Scarry's seminal *The Body in Pain* highlights the difficulty in sharing the experience of pain in that it resists objectification in language (1985, 5). There are no words that can completely and accurately share the felt intensity of pain. Likewise, the felt experience of lived experiences of recovery from addiction resist translation into spoken word. Artistic expression, however, assists through its liminal state to generate a valence of feeling that might better express the texture of these lived experiences. In the Repair Centre project, objects were the storytellers. They claimed agency in becoming the narrators of a display of experiences of trauma, healing and acceptance.

The objects collated for the Repair Centre offered an eclectic exhibition including an otherwise conventional-looking blue check shirt sporting a newly attached paisley print collar, a series of coasters upcycled from broken branches and cutlery with newly acquired paper pulp handles. The oddity of this assemblage invites us to consider what we might learn from unconventional forms of repair; that recovery from addiction – or reconstruction in the context of the project – does not follow a pre-set pattern. Nonetheless, the divergence of these objects from the conventional gestures towards an appreciation of the complex and varied lived experiences of recovery.

Performance as Agonistic Activism

It is appropriate, and often evident, that recovery-engaged arts practice addresses the features of tension and conflict that are encountered during (and prior to) processes of recovery. These features entail the personal and societal factors that impact upon different people differently. I proposed in Chapter 2 that, through their struggle with addiction and practices of recovery, people in recovery are particularly aware of their own antagonistic relationship with their surroundings. By revealing counter-narratives, representations different to predominant notions of the 'addict' identity, the examples of artistry included in this chapter perform in accordance to Mouffe's concept of 'radical democracy' (2013, 7). They operate as a form of agonistic activism by not only 'making visible' (93) that which has often been obscured, but also by enabling a localised pluralist democracy through cultural participation. Performers, artists, participants-in-recovery can, therefore, claim active citizenship within recovery-engaged creative communities.

Continuing my emphasis on the nonhuman dimension of these arts practices, I extend Ahmed's discussion of 'sticky affect' (2010, 29) to consider how the 'addict' body in its circulation in society becomes an object to which certain pejorative, and marginalising, stereotypes become attached. Recovery-engaged arts practices hold the potential to reveal, challenge and, perhaps, subvert the context-specific 'affective economies' (Ahmed 2014, 8) that hinder capacities for recovery by confining people in recovery to associations of deviant or unvalued citizenship.

Affective Economies of the 'Addict Identity'

Too High Too Far Too Soon raises awareness of the hypocritical values of western society. Much of Mason's story is placed within the social context of the British music industry of the late 1980s and 1990s. The narrative reveals the less glamourous aspects of festival and gig culture that are usually associated with celebrity. For instance, in the scene we entitled 'Knebworth – Happy Birthday Smackhead', Mason, who is by then in an entrenched state of active addiction to heroin, re-enacts a moment from a toilet cubicle amid the exclusive backstage area of a high-profile concert. During this scene, Mason is suffering from withdrawal symptoms and has discovered that he has lost the heroin he brought with him. Frantically searching for the missing 'baggie' of heroin he strips to his underpants. Alone, and desperate, the action culminates with him crying and shaking in the cubicle. Two scenes later, the audience view another toilet setting, this time at a music industry promotional party that Mason has been given responsibility for organising on the premise that he will provide free cocaine for the guests. On discovering that the guest list has grown to a size much bigger than he was prepared for, or able to fund, Mason spends the evening hiding in the toilet using his supply of drugs by himself. While this performance was agonistic in revealing the underbelly of an industry better known for its glamorous lifestyle, I suggest that the political potential of this performance was the way in which economies of social value, or 'affective economies' (Ahmed 2014, 8), were revealed.

Ahmed's 'affective economies' provide a useful approach to examining the milieu of addiction created in the artistic practices discussed in this chapter. She proposed that 'feelings' do not 'reside' in people or objects, but that they are 'produced as effects of their circulation' (2014, 8). I interpret her discussion to suggest that we can deduce the hierarchies of value that operate in society by observing the patterns of emotion that are projected onto certain bodies or objects. By refusing to attribute the cause of the emotion to the person or thing under observation, we can address the sociopolitical influences that inform what are considered to be social 'norms'. Ahmed's examination of the political consequences of affective economies is particularly relevant to my discussion in demonstrating how they function to reinforce hegemonic norms and exclude those who do not conform. If our cultural worlds are constructed by 'feeling our way' (12), then it is useful to attend to how certain feelings are associated with people affected by addiction and how this impacts on their sociability in society.

The Repair Centre objects intervene in existing affective economies by disrupting normative values of brokenness. They remind us that repair is possible and, most importantly, that repair need not conform to conventional ideas of 'becoming well'. Reflecting on efforts towards decoloniality, Mischa Twitchin highlights the fallacy of western acts of repair aimed at the disappearance of the wound (2021, 54). For Twitchin, it is the coexistence of break and mend that truly transforms the integrity of the object of repair. Denial of the past impedes meaningful progress. Like their metamorphosed object, participants in the Repair Centre project do not deny their past. They take account of it, while committing to a process of transformation.

The critical visibility of *Too High Too Far Too Soon* and the Repair Centre is formed by the way in which the nonhuman contributors reveal the systemic economies that constitute the milieu of an addicted person and, subsequently, inform the identities they come to inhabit. By systemic, I refer to the structures of society, institutional operations and cultural practices that perpetuate certain norms and hierarchies. I suggest that it is these systemic features that can hinder capacity for recovery, reminding us that 'becoming well' (Duff 2016, 58) requires an environment in which interdependency and collective support are valued. As Bennett's vital materialism highlights, we are all interconnected in the greater ecology of things in the world (2010, 13). I suggest that the examples discussed here offer an opportunity to review the way in which these connections operate. What values are revealed when we look at how 'addict' bodies and associated objects circulate in society? What feelings, or 'sticky affects' (Ahmed 2014, 11), are attributed to these objects as a consequence of their circulation in society? I am particularly interested in how recovery-engaged performances might reveal and then challenge these sticky affects.

In *Too High Too Far Too Soon* the 'sticky' objects associated with Mason's life, discussed earlier, might evoke emotive responses that reveal our 'affective forms of reorientation' towards or away from these objects which in turn demonstrates the values they have acquired respective to the contingent contexts of their circulation in society (Ahmed 2014). If we also consider the body as an object in correlation with these items associated with addiction and that lifestyle, it is possible to explore the affective economy in which they exist. As Ahmed states in her discussion of 'Happy Objects', normative bodies and objects conform to societal notions of what is deemed 'good' (2010, 41). Those that deviate from social norms are deemed to be the cause of bad affect as they fail to take part in the happiness of the experience of the majority. They become, what Ahmed has coined, 'affect aliens' (37). In *The Cultural Politics of Emotion* (2014), Ahmed developed this argument to demonstrate how bodies of black, Asian or global majority ethnicities, particularly the feminine, become objects of hate or disgust in the way in which their presence disrupts social hierarchies founded on male whiteness (4 and 58). Drug policies associated with the War on Drugs, and much of the media representation of addiction in contemporary society, generates an affective economy in which most addicts become positioned as 'embodied deviants', objects of hate and disgust (Ettorre 2015, 6). Positioning the experience of addiction as attached to deviant bodies deflects from critical reflection on the systemic issues that fuel addiction as a coping strategy for survival. Mason's autobiographical story highlights the societal contradictions that reify celebrity and wealth without addressing the counter-consequences that occur when money and fame are prioritised over ethical forms of interaction.

The hypocrisy of the differentiated affective economies within drug-using circles is also revealed in *Too High Too Far Too Soon* to demonstrate the hierarchies in operation that privilege certain bodies and addictive behaviours over others. For instance, Mason attained status and subsequent pleasure as a cocaine and ecstasy dealer and user within the Britpop social circle in the 1990s. Once his growing heroin addiction became apparent, he became an object of disgust and was gradually excluded from that circle. The juxtapositions discussed earlier of toilet settings in what would otherwise be considered as glamorous celebrity settings highlights the differing status of the recreational cocaine user versus the addicted heroin user. We are reminded that across society exist microcosms of differentiated social economies in which certain forms of addiction are considered more tolerable than others. Conversely, the Repair Centre offers an approach to reclaiming social value through demonstrating aesthetically that what was once considered broken can be transformed.

Conclusion

The performance of *Too High Too Far Too Soon* and the Repair Centre participatory art project presented an assemblage of experiences of addiction and recovery. By emphasising the ways in which objects operated in each project, I highlight the potential of reading them as material constellations that reveal the complex milieus that influence different realities of addiction and recovery. As indicated by posthumanist addiction research, by attending to the nonhuman aspects of experience – and the manner in which these collide with the human – we might better understand the varied factors that create the 'normality' of someone affected by addiction (Dennis and Farrugia 2017, 1) or that inhibit capacity for 'becoming well' (Duff 2016, 58). By decentring the human through my emphasis on the nonhuman contributors, I underscore the contingent and systemic features of the experiences shared and, therefore, reveal the potential for recovery-engaged arts to contribute to a more nuanced understanding of addiction and recovery.

For future practice, work with objects might assist with developing further the potential of generating spaces of potentiality in arts practices that are engaged with the lived realities of addiction and recovery. It is pertinent, however, to also understand the ethical complexity of engaging with 'sticky' objects that might evoke addiction-based sensations. Such forms of practice are contingent on the recovery practices and relations of care in operation within given spaces and places.

Notes

1 Performed by Denise Gough, the lead character Emma is an actor who, now in rehab, struggles with her treatment programme. Her resistance to the process and conflictual interactions with others there reveal the difficulties of recovery from addiction. The play places emphasis on her journey towards personal accountability, however, and does not, in my view, fully explore the other contextual factors that influence her addiction-based coping strategies. Specifically, the co-dependent dynamic of Emma's relationship with her mother is briefly revealed as problematic towards the end of play, but is left undeveloped.
2 At the time of this project, I was Artistic Director of Outside Edge Theatre Company. Due to the sudden death of my colleague and founder of the company, Phil

Fox, I had been promoted from Associate to Artistic Director in June 2014 and assumed responsibility for completing the directorial projects he had been contracted to undertake that year. I use this example of prior practice as an exemplar for discussion rather than practice research as my theoretical analysis is retrospective rather than emerging simultaneous to doing the practice.

3 Neurological research on the impact of long-term heavy drug use on the brain indicates that 'chronic abuse of drugs may impact directly on neural memory systems' causing dysfunction (Robbins et al. 2008). A study by Cadet and Bisagno (2016) identified the forms of cognitive impairment caused by abuse of certain drugs such as marijuana, cocaine and methamphetamine. Impairment of memory was identified in each case.

4 Marlatt and Donovan acknowledge in the introduction to their book *Relapse Prevention* that factors influencing relapse are 'idiosyncratic' and 'fluctuating' (2005, 3). They propose that relapse prevention is enhanced by the learning of self-management skills and maintaining a lifestyle balance that reduces stressors.

5 We broke the solo performance down into scenes that could be isolated for rehearsal but also assisted recall and were directly related to an object and a location in the performance space.

6 Detox refers to the stage when clients in a treatment programme are undergoing withdrawal from addictive substances. During this phase of vulnerability, they may experience symptoms of physical illness, emotional extremes and a strong urge to use their addictive substance.

7 A series of blogs documenting the creative workshops of the Repair Centre can be found on PORe's website: https://portraitsofrecovery.org.uk/news/kintsugi-inspired-ceramic-reconstructions/#.

References

Ahmed, S. (2010) 'Happy objects', in M. Gregg and G.J. Seigworth (eds), *The affect theory reader*. Durham, NC: Duke University Press, pp. 29–50.

Ahmed, S. (2014) *The cultural politics of emotion*. 2nd ed. Edinburgh: Edinburgh University Press.

Barad, K. (2008) 'Posthumanist performativity: Towards an understanding of how matter comes to matter', in S. Alaimo and S. Hekman (eds), *Material feminisms*. Bloomington: Indiana University Press, pp. 120–154.

Bennett, J. (2010) *Vibrant matter: A political ecology of things*. Durham, NC: Duke University Press.

Berlant, L. (2010) 'Cruel optimism', in M. Gregg and G.J. Seigworth (eds), *The affect theory reader*. Durham, NC: Duke University Press, pp. 94–117.

Bernstein, R. (2009) 'Dances with things', *Social Text*, 27 (4), pp. 67–94. Available at: https://doi.org/10.1215/01642472-2009-055.

Cadet, J.L. and Bisagno, V. (2016) 'Neuropsychological consequences of chronic drug use: Relevance to treatment approaches', *Frontiers in Psychiatry*, 6. Available at: https://doi.org/10.3389/fpsyt.2015.00189.

Dennis, F. and Farrugia, A. (2017) 'Materialising drugged pleasures: Practice, politics, care', *International Journal of Drug Policy*, 49, pp. 86–91.

Dobkin, P.L. (2022) 'Kintsugi mind: How clinicians can be restored rather than broken by the pandemic', *Canadian Family Physician*, 68 (4), pp. 252–254. Available at: https://doi.org/10.46747/cfp.6804252.

Duff, C. (2014) *Assemblages of health: Deleuze's empiricism and the ethology of life*. New York: Springer.

Duff, C. (2016) 'Atmospheres of recovery: Assemblages of health', *Environment and Planning A*, 48 (1), pp. 58–74. Available at: https://doi.org/10.1177/0308518X15603222.

Eckersall, P. and Grehan, H. (2021) 'Necessity or choice: Demanding the right to repair', *Performance Research*, 26 (6), pp. 1–4. Available at: https://doi.org/10.1080/13528165.2021.2059158.

Ettorre, E. (2015) 'Embodied deviance, gender, and epistemologies of ignorance: Re-visioning drugs use in a neurochemical, unjust world', *Substance Use & Misuse*, 50 (6), pp. 794–805. Available at: https://doi.org/10.3109/10826084.2015.978649.

Harpin, A. (2018) *Madness, art, and society: Beyond illness*. London and New York: Routledge.

Harris, A.M. and Holman Jones, S.L. (2019) *The queer life of things: Performance, affect, and the more-than-human*. Lanham, MD: Lexington Books.

Kemske, B. (2021) *Kintsugi: The poetic mend*. London: Herbert Press.

Lewis, M.D. (2016) *The biology of desire: Why addiction is not a disease*. Melbourne and London: Scribe Publications.

Macmillan, D. (2015) *People, places and things*. London: Oberon Books.

Marlatt, G.A. and Donovan, D.M. (eds) (2005) *Relapse prevention: Maintenance strategies in the treatment of addictive behaviors*. 2nd ed. New York: Guilford Press.

Mason, S. (2013) *Too high, too far, too soon: Tales from a dubious past*. Edinburgh: Mainstream Publishing.

Mayo, S. (n.d.) 'Interview with Rachel Ho', *Breaks and Joins*. Available at: http://www.suemayo.co.uk/breaks-and-joins-podcasts/.

Moten, F. and Harney, S. (2013) *The undercommons: Fugitive planning & black study*. Wivenhoe: Minor Compositions.

Mouffe, C. (2013) *Agonistics: Thinking the world politically*. London and New York: Verso.

O'Grady, A. (ed.) (2017) *Risk, participation, and performance practice*. New York: Palgrave Macmillan.

Robbins, T.W., Ersche, K.D. and Everitt, B.J. (2008) 'Drug addiction and the memory systems of the brain', *Annals of the New York Academy of Sciences*, 1141 (1), pp. 1–21. Available at: https://doi.org/10.1196/annals.1441.020.

Scarry, E. (1985) *The body in pain: The making and unmaking of the world*. New York: Oxford University Press.

Selman, L. (2021) 'Covid grief has cracked us open: How clinicians respond could reshape attitudes to bereavement – An essay by Lucy Selman', *BMJ*, p. 1803. Available at: https://doi.org/10.1136/bmj.n1803.

Twitchin, M. (2021) 'On repair: Between cosmopolitics and decoloniality', *Performance Research*, 26 (6), pp. 54–61. Available at: https://doi.org/10.1080/13528165.2021.2059162.

Zontou, Z. (2014) 'Staging recovery from addiction', in J. Reynolds and Z. Zontou (eds), *Addiction and performance*. Newcastle upon Tyne: Cambridge Scholars Publishing, pp. 338–357.

Zontou, Z. (2017) 'Upon awakening: Addiction, performance, and aesthetics of authenticity', in A. O'Grady (ed.), *Risk, participation, and performance practice: Critical vulnerabilities in a precarious world*. New York: Palgrave Macmillan, pp. 205–231.

4 Place in Recovery-Engaged Performance

'Context is everything', claim Kelly Freebody and Michael Finneran in their discussion of the role of place in community drama projects (2021, 83). This chapter examines the importance of local and global ideas of place in recovery-engaged performance practice, particularly how reimagining relationships with place can contribute to atmospheres of recovery. Place and time are not static or singular. As Freebody and Finneran point out, the place-time of the performance event is a fluid, cross-temporal entity with the potential to traverse the local and global as well as to create 'alternative public spaces' through which participants might redefine their relationship within a given place or community (89).

The context of experiences of addiction and recovery is composed of complex and varied assemblages of the human and nonhuman features of any given moment of life. For Duff, understanding how bodies, spaces, affects and relations assemble in the event of drug use enables a more accurate appreciation of the subjectivities of addiction, including how the more-than-human elements impact lived experience (2014, 127). Often this includes geographical location and the prevailing cultural or legislative codes that inform how those affected by addiction are classified and managed within systems of health, social policy or criminal justice. Performances on stage and screen have portrayed the geo-historical contexts of waves of addiction. For instance, Ed Edwards' play *The Political History of Smack and Crack* (2018) situates the chaotic antics of two addicts, Mandy and Neil, amid the wave of heroin addiction that emerged in Manchester, UK, in the early 1980s. Using humour and pathos, the audience is guided through the literal highs and lows of the two characters. It is the socio-economic setting of the play, however, that conveys the key message that Edwards wishes to share. In an addendum to the printed play text, Edwards correlates the rise of the 'hard drug epidemic' across the UK with the spread of Thatcherite neoliberal economic policy (71). Poverty and social deprivation, exacerbated by an unprecedented rise in unemployment, are framed as the context of the drug using assemblages of Mandy and Neil and countless others within working-class communities of that era.

Edwards also offers, in this addendum, a summary of the international politics that form the macro-level milieu of the rise of the hard drug epidemic

DOI: 10.4324/9781003271062-5

involving CIA-sponsored narcotic trade to fund US- and UK-backed counter-revolutionary insurgents in Nicaragua and Afghanistan, respectively, in the 1980s (2018, 89 and 90). The theme of intelligence service collusion with drug trafficking and its subsequent contribution to the rise in hard drug addiction is also portrayed in the long-running American television series, *Snowfall* (FX 2017–). This series not only correlates addiction with poverty, but also demonstrates the added influences of systemic racism and social injustice that formed the backdrop of the crack cocaine epidemic in South Central Los Angeles, USA, in the 1980s. Both *The Political History of Smack and Crack* and *Snowfall* demonstrate the potential of performance to simultaneously reveal the localised idiosyncrasies of geographically located experience of addiction as well as the ways in which the global milieu merges with the local. Freebody and Finneran offer an understanding of this merger of global and local as a 'circular process' by which they comprehend drama as 'not only informed by global issues or attending to local issues' but as a combination of the two conceived as 'glocalisation' (2021, 81). Given the influence of international policy and trade on drugs, whether legal or illicit, recovery-engaged performances are especially attuned to glocal dynamics that can fuel addiction and inhibit recovery.

The encounters with recovery-engaged theatre practice discussed in this chapter highlight the ways in which performance can reveal, subvert and reimagine ideas of place in relation to the experience of being in recovery. First, the example of Sonya Hale's *Like Butterflies* is offered as an illustration of how a performance text written by someone with lived experience of addiction recovery presents a differing perspective of the site-specific features of street dwelling and challenges hierarchies of social value in relation to the bodily experiences of street drug users. To highlight the glocal politics of *Like Butterflies*, I discuss how the creation and performance of this work occurred in relation to the international milieu of the #MeToo movement in 2017–2018. Second, I share my experience of Outside Edge Theatre Company's Open House event in 2018 to examine the 'messy connections' with place, recovery community and performance activity that contribute to the milieu in which the organisation operates. My reference to place in this instance specifically focuses on 61 Munster Road, a house in Fulham, West London, UK, that had been converted into an addiction treatment facility and was also Outside Edge's base from 1998–2020. The glocal features of this example resonate with the rise of austerity measures and subsequent cuts to public funding of addiction services emerging from the continued impact of the global economic recession from 2008 onwards.

Ideas of Place

Massey's concepts of space are influential to my understanding of place in this chapter. Given that space is always under construction through interrelations with the human, the nonhuman and the temporal, it is useful for performance practice to also consider place as a space that is multiple, plural and constantly evolving. It is 'a simultaneity of stories so far' (2005, 9). Recovery-engaged performance practice can reveal and interrogate these stories, potentially offering new narratives. Place, then, might be conceived as the momentary location of space within a given geographic, temporal and social milieu. Constructed through affective interactions with the human and the nonhuman, Massey reminds us that these interactions are very likely conflictual and unequal (153). By framing place as a negotiation, Massey reveals its democratic potential through attending to the ways in which social relations construct it (155–156).

Mackey's extensive applied theatre research on place practices offers a useful guide to approaching place as 'always already temporary' (2016, 110). By recognising place as constructed through temporary, inter-relational experience, she conceives the local as constituted by periods of dwelling (110). Mackey's reference to dwelling resonates with the examples of recovery-engaged performance discussed below in that both *Like Butterflies* and the Open House event reveal differing experiences of familiarity and habitation in the respective located spaces entailed in these examples. Performance practice can disrupt set ideas about place and construct new narratives as such activity 'identifies, makes explicit, interrogates and shifts or alters relationships with place' (107). It can also resist normative assumptions of place and dwelling, which is especially useful for drawing attention to located assemblages of addiction and recovery.

Subverting Associations with Place

The narrative of *Like Butterflies* begins at an illegal rave, in a barn, at an undisclosed location somewhere in the English countryside. The protagonist of this solo performance, Shelly, exudes joyful excitement as she shares her memory of her visceral interactions within this temporary habitation of the rural by urban beats and bodies. We are presented with a Halberstamian 'queer subject' (Massey 2005, 10) for whom norms of time, place, gendered behaviour and linguistic vernacular are suspended in the underworld of rave culture in the early 1990s. Shelley awakens from where she lost consciousness beside a bass bin speaker to discover she has been handcuffed to a stranger in a prank by friends. The first music track of the performance plays, Crazy Town's rap rock single 'My Butterfly', and the hedonistic revelry begins.

> I hear that fit beat twanging … I leap to my feet and yank him.
> 'Oi that hurts', he says, but I give it, 'I fucking love this tune mate, innit! Fucking yes! Fucking 'avin it! Love it!'
> And we dance handcuffed together … *(Tune starts to fade…)*
> And I don't care we don't give a fuck of flying about the handcuffs, we are just airborne innit. And then we like run, give it legs,

> We leave behind the party, all those wickle-ickle-mummy-boys and all their girlfriends in their sad, sad world, everyone dance to the same old tune, same old fucking tune and we run out, out, out, so far out … To these fields of corn and it is like spikey but…[1]

Like Butterflies is a piece of writing for the stage that was commissioned by producer Ellie Keel for the Alchemy theatre festival (North Wall Arts Centre, Oxford, UK, 6–8 April 2018). My discussion focuses on the way in which objects featured in the scripted text of the monologue to evoke an imagined assemblage of a specific, contextualised experience of addiction. Their 'vital materialism' (Bennett 2010, 12) emanated through their use as devices to evoke place, setting and time, specifically the situated experience of a young woman whose life is affected by homelessness, addiction and assault. These operate as an imagined constellation that reveals the 'milieu' – the located environment – that constructs the 'addict' identity of the narrative's protagonist, Shelly.

My discussion draws on the monologue text used for rehearsal, my viewing of the piece in performance at the Alchemy theatre festival, and a recorded conversation with the writer, Sonya Hale. As noted in the Introduction to this volume, my position as a practitioner within the small field of recovery arts in the UK has assisted my access to the creative process of other artists and practitioners mentioned in this book. In this instance, I note that I have a prior history of working with Hale in my capacity as a practitioner with Outside Edge Theatre. She began as a participant in 2011, progressing to writing for stage apprenticeship and, by 2014, had become a workshop facilitator. Having followed her progress as a professionally commissioned writer, I am able to draw on a particular insight into the development of her artistic work, including access to unpublished writing such as the text of *Like Butterflies*. Hale unfortunately died of cancer in November 2020, marking an abrupt end to her brief career as a professional playwright. Nonetheless, she leaves a legacy of unique play texts that offer insights informed by her own immersion in spaces and places of addiction and, subsequently, recovery.

Informed by Hale's own embodied knowledge of addiction and recovery, *Like Butterflies* communicates the materiality of the non-normative world of a homeless teenager who is also a habitual drug user. It provides a specifically gendered and class experience of a young woman from a working-class background. The main character, Shelly, a 'twenty-something woman with a broad northern English accent', shares with the audience a story about her experience of street dwelling at the age of sixteen. Hale combines the description of bodily action and mundane objects that creates an image of bodily deviance from usual social norms and a sense of the material conditions in which it is situated. Her use of language is purposefully emotive, indicating a particular affective relation with other people, places and things. The vernacular of Shelly blends northern dialect with patterns of multicultural London English, denoting a linguistic assemblage influenced by the different social cultures that contribute to the transitory worlds that the protagonist inhabits. Hale invites us to view the imagined constellation from Shelly's perspective, rather than our own. We enter a space of potentiality in which we might discover a new, or revised, understanding of the located experience shared with us.

Disrupting Stereotypes of Place and the 'Dangerous Other'

(Content warning: the latter part of this section contains references to experience of sexual violence.)

Isabel Lorey's concept of the 'dangerous other' (2015, 38) is particularly relevant to the position of the 'addict' within societal contexts whereby government policy is still bound tightly to the politics of prohibition and criminalisation of drug use. Her proposition that the *affect* of fear is utilised as an instrument of control by government systems (2) reinforces Ettorre's analysis that addicts are often stigmatised and marginalised by being regarded by mainstream society as 'embodied deviants' (2015, 6). To some extent fear might be considered a natural defence mechanism for human and animal beings; however, it can also result in exclusion and blame. As Lorey suggests, when faced with uncertainty, people strive to reduce their vulnerability through compliance to the hegemonic norm, i.e. that which is considered to be normal or good citizenship within a given political regime (2015, 26–29). 'Addicts', therefore, become 'dangerous others' in their failure to conform within the prevailing norm. Marginalisation and stigmatisation are, therefore, the consequential experience of bodies labelled as 'affect aliens' (Ahmed 2010, 50) by their noncompliance upon which is projected the fear and disgust of those aspiring to the ideal norm. This 'alien' biopolitical position can be used to justify harsher policies that further criminalise addicted people. For instance, the incumbent UK Conservative government's White Paper consultation, *Swift, Certain, Tough: New Consequences for Drug Possession* (HMSO 2022) proposes a significant escalation of penalties for people caught in possession of recreational drugs. Tier three of the proposed sanctions includes possible confiscation of the offender's passport, drive licence disqualification, an exclusion order and tagging.

The opening of Hale's *Like Butterflies*, shared above, defiantly emphasises joyfulness and camaraderie amid the chaos and resistance to a normative lifestyle. I do not consider this moment as intended to glorify drug use. Instead, it is consistent with Hale's agenda to challenge hegemonic values implicit in how working-class and non-normative lifestyles, such as drug users, rough sleepers or criminal offenders, are represented on stage and on screen. In an interview for Arcola Theatre, she expressed her concern that working-class lives should not be portrayed as bleak and horrible when, in her experience, there is 'so much creativity and laughter and beauty and heart'.[2] Hale is certainly not the first to use theatre to challenge the representation of such lifestyles. Companies such as Clean Break, Cardboard Citizens and Synergy, to name but a few within the sphere of applied theatre, specialise in commissioning new work that reveals counter-narratives to the stereotypes that have marginalised those affected by homelessness, the criminal justice system and substance dependency.

Kate Beswick's performance research on representations of the working-class council estate highlights how socially engaged performance can subvert the dominant narratives and stereotypes to 'demonstrate a form of spatial critique' (2011, 434).[3] Performance as a spatial practice can, therefore, be harnessed as a powerful tool through which those often excluded from the dominant academic and social discourses can intervene by creating alternative representations (434). In the following excerpt, for example, Hale provides the audience with an alternative perspective of the site-specific features of an urban rough sleeper's dwelling.

> And down this alley at the back of Tesco, down this snug cush-up alley, we get cardboard boxes, mattress, blankets, we make a wooden roof and everything and cover it in bubble wrap innit. Our little home and it's like nearly waterproof and everyfin, our little home, *our skipper* and we are so snuggly tuck up in there innit.

Mundane objects – that are in fact discarded refuse items – are lovingly arranged by Shelly and her partner 'T' to create a home. Rather than considering this improvised accommodation as debased, in the way that those of us privileged with no experience of homelessness might instinctively respond, we are offered the opportunity to engage in a new affective relation with these items. During my own encounter with this section of the performance, I felt a new relation with the objects described above from their contextualisation as demonstrating love and care, as evoking sensations of belonging and comfort.

The domesticity of this scene also emphasises a gendered association with Shelly as a teenage woman who, in the narrative, takes comfort in the protection that her boyfriend T provides. The first half of the monologue follows a theme of love and romance, although with the promise of gender equality in how they operate as a team in creating their home and 'grafting'[4] for the means to buy food and drugs. The idealism of this domestic arrangement is suddenly disrupted by a traumatic incident which Hale uses as a mechanism to highlight the specifically gendered experience of female street dwellers. In particular, she intended to spotlight the experience of violence against women, whose stories, she argued, are not as visible as other examples of gender violence.

In the extract below Shelly describes her experience of sexual assault that unravels the narrative of the initial love story. As before, the description of inorganic objects is used to create a detailed impression of the material experience of the event. Shelly and T have developed a routine whereby she lures men into their 'cush-up' alley so that he can rob them and so acquire enough money to feed their growing drug consumption. The moment described below is when the plan unravels with traumatic consequences for Shelly.

And finally a man stops in his van, non-descript, white van man ... he gets out, dark hair I think, normal, and I take him down the back alley, down the back of Tesco innit. Down *our alley*, the place where our skipper is and T, said he promised, he promised he'd be there waiting ... But when we get there I can't see him and I think shit, shit, shit ... (Beat) I ask him for the fucking money innit? I do ask him but he won't fucking give it to me. Cunt. He just pulls down his trousers and ... (Beat) ... I start shouting loud for T but he grabs my face and he pushes me. He pushes me and pushes me, hard up against the back wall innit. (Beat) And all I can feel is my body scraping, scratching, scrunched on the rough concrete ... (Beat).

And when the man leaves, when he has finished I swear down he thanks me ... He chucks me twenty quid and he like leaves me there on the concrete ... Just walks away.

The image of concrete as an aggressive actant emerges from this part of the performed narrative. Not only in its abrasiveness to Shelly's skin, but also through Hale's description of how, in the following weeks after this event, it sucks away the vibrant colours of the autumnal environment to a 'cold, hard, relentless grey' (6). The joyfulness has been arrested, so too the love narrative culminating in the arrest of T and his incarceration by the police for theft, leaving Shelly abandoned in what has become reframed as a harsh, bleak environment. This section of the monologue reveals the conflictual ways in which bodies, objects and place collide painfully in such lived experiences. Moreover, the discomfort I felt on hearing it, at a point in time when discussions related to #MeToo and #NoGreyArea were fresh, caused me to reflect that not all women's experiences are treated with equal compassion.

It is useful to note here the following key events from the global sociopolitical milieu in which *Like Butterflies* was written and performed. From October 2017, the previous year, when allegations of sexual harassment were publicly revealed against Hollywood film producer Harvey Weinstein, responses to this event proliferated into a worldwide, viral campaign (#MeToo and #TimesUp) to raise awareness of and support for the victims of sexual violence in the workplace, particularly in the entertainment industry. In the UK, Vicky Featherstone, Artistic Director of the Royal Court Theatre, organised the #NoGreyArea campaign, a series of events encouraging the sharing of experiences that culminated in the formulation of a set of guidelines for the British theatre industry on how to establish working practices that prevent instances of sexual harassment. During 2017 and 2018, there were a vast array of initiatives online from feminist activists to challenge the persistent existence of harassment of women.[5] It is also important to note that the term #MeToo was appropriated from its original use by activist Tarana Burke who initially employed the phrase to promote the empowerment of women of black and global majority heritages who have experienced sexual abuse. Its uptake by a celebrity-initiated mainstream social media movement highlights the contradictory values of care that Hale chose to address in her writing. In a conversation with me at the time she was in the process of writing *Like Butterflies* she indicated that this new piece of work was her contribution to the #MeToo debate.

Like Butterflies particularly drew attention to the contradictions of the milieu of the #MeToo campaign in which hierarchies of value and care operate, rendering some bodies as beyond the social norm and, therefore, deviant. Shelly's narrative depicts the harsh, grey and mundane reality of the material conditions of some women, street dwellers or others marginalised by poverty. In conversation, Hale revealed her commitment to highlighting this social injustice when writing the monologue.

> When I was homeless, there was this kind of feeling that sexual violence happens to you, it's just what happens. Y'know like, yeah, it's upsetting, but you just kind of crack on with it. And it was almost like a completely different class of crime to sexual violence happening to a 'normal' person.

Hale is not, of course, the first writer to challenge the hypocrisy of how the experiences of certain bodies are privileged over others. Here, the materiality of Hale's narrative of Shelly serves as a reminder of the sociocultural circumstances, marking some women as less deserving of compassion, that contribute to assemblages of addiction. Compassion may well be associated with capacity for empathy. Carolyn Pedwell's discussion of the affective process of empathy as 'a social and political relation' aligns with Ahmed's affective economies in that empathetic relation is generated by feelings that are produced as effects of a body's or object's circulation within a given social context (2014, xi). Empathy is uneven, contingent and differently felt across cultural and geopolitical contexts (3). Drawing on Berlant's politics of emotion, Pedwell notes that empathy and compassion are bound up by ethics of privilege (15). Ambivalence, or a withholding of compassionate feeling, denotes power and privilege in the refusal to engage or care. Pedwell, while emphasising that ideas of empathy can be harnessed by neoliberal governmentality in ways that reinforce pervading social injustices, suggests that 'radical intersections of empathy, hope and imagination' can operate as 'an affective portal to different spaces and times' where the nature of empathy can be negotiated (46).

Hale's re-representation of the features of place stimulated opportunities to also re-evaluate the felt spectrum of empathy, moving the spectator from ambivalence to fellow feeling. Specifically, *Like Butterflies* invites us to adopt an agonistic approach to compassion. This continues my application of Mouffe's ideas about agonism (2013, 93) in the previous chapter to examine how performance can create an 'aesthetics of critical visibility' (Fisher 2017, 20) that not only reveals underrepresented experience but also highlights the power structures that impact on lived experience. Shelly is poor, living on the street, on the margins of what might be considered an acceptable lifestyle by mainstream society. She engages in activities such as theft and illicit drug use which are likely to incur negative judgement from some people and are illegal.

Although she does not engage in sex work in this narrative, her ruse to lure men into the alleyway to be robbed by T alludes to this activity. As Julia Downes' article for *The Conversation* about the limits of the #MeToo campaign noted that 'not all women are safe to speak out' (2018). Downes argued that, based on her research on criminology and social policy, the working practices of the current legal systems in the US and the UK at ground level are likely to result in the arrest of victims rather than the conviction of their abusers (2018).

Hale's depiction of the visceral, bodily attributes of Shelly's experience challenges us to move beyond ambivalence or at least, during the sensorial exchange of the performance, to feel something alongside the protagonist. I suggest that the narrative attempts to achieve this by emphasising Shelly's bodily experience of physical pain and psychological hurt within the familiar location of a bathroom shower; a common and yet private place that quickly connotes a sense of intimacy with the audience. In particular, the excerpt below draws attention to the materiality of Shelly's body through its relation with bathroom objects and water. It also hints towards shared bodily knowledge of practices of self-care and cleansing that have the potential to resonate with the other human bodies viewing the performance. In this excerpt, Shelly has been brought into a homeless shelter and has her first shower since the sexual assault some weeks ago.

> Down at the centre they tell me I need a shower innit. I say fuck off but they say I've got bad nits and I am itchy and I got foot rot. They hand me like a scrubbing brush thing and a bar of soap and a towel … I head into the shower and I peel off my clothes. (Beat) It dawns on me I ain't … Not since …
>
> I get in the shower. Turn on the hot tap … I feel it … (Beat)
>
> It burns. I let it burn me … and then I wash and wash and scrub and scrub. I mean, I have seen women on tele do this so I know what the fuck I'm doing, I ain't stupid but I just can't help it, I keep scrubbing and scrubbing and scrubbing till I am red raw hurting and then I sit down in the shower for what feels like ages … and I watch it all drain away … all skin and dirt and bubbles.

The political potential of Shelly's narrative resides in its capacity for making critically visible aspects of societal experience that are uncomfortable and challenging in how they reveal the inequities of how some experiences, and some people, are attributed less value than others. We are challenged to feel compassion for Shelly, someone who might not otherwise be afforded such a relation of care within a society that often renders 'addicts' as deviant and criminal and where public comfort is found in distancing these experiences from what is considered normal society, denying them visibility. *Like Butterflies* reminds the audience that, although different and engaged in activities that might be unfamiliar or undesirable to those watching, Shelly experiences the affective spectrum of joy, pleasure, pain and loss, to which many people can relate.

Like Butterflies reveals the conflictual affective economy in which Shelley's body operates. Ahmed's discussion of the experience of pain particularly demonstrated how affectivity forms the human body as 'both a material and lived entity (2014, 24). The body might, therefore, be conceived as a material object *and* an experience of being. In the narrative of *Like Butterflies,* Shelly's body was presented as simultaneously an object associated with fun, tenderness and love, that also experiences violence, disgust and rejection. Quite literally, at one point, it becomes attached with dirt, sweat and blood. Shelly is an 'affect alien', although one particularly impacted by the implications of gender politics revealed through the way in which her partner T withdraws from her after she is raped by the stranger he was supposed to rob. Blame for her own trauma is implicit in both the narrative and T's initial accusation that she 'let him do it'. Through the emotive experience of listening to Shelly's story, we are invited to connect affectively to the body her character represents. I might assume, for most present during the live performance in a comfortable arts venue in Oxford, that the narrative presented was different to most of the audience's own lived experience. Nonetheless, in revealing the shared humanity in our capacity to be affected by love and pain, we might be challenged to re-evaluate societal assumptions that privilege some bodies over others, that might otherwise dehumanise Shelly's 'deviant' body as beyond compassion.

The absence of mechanisms of support for Shelly in the narrative also infers the systemic inequalities that exist in relation to support provision for victims of sexual violence, and more generally, gender-specific recovery needs. As Campbell and Ettorre pointed out in *Gendering Addiction*, despite efforts since the 1970s to improve treatment services available to women, drug treatment in the US and the UK is still delivered in ways with which many cannot engage (2014, 1). They argue that women, and also people from other marginalised groups, are unable to access effective support due to 'epistemologies of ignorance' that neglect gendered, classed and racialised power differentials (1). Their research endorsed the creation of new knowledges, using methods that could acknowledge absent voices and embrace the multidimensional and emotional, or I would argue the *affective*, narratives of lived experience. I suggest that *Like Butterflies*, and other such performances, can contribute to these new knowledges. Socially engaged arts have the capacity to reveal insights into everyday experience that, if acknowledged by researchers in addiction treatment, could contribute to the creation of more astutely tailored approaches to programmes of recovery support.

Hale's representation of alternative narratives of place in *Like Butterflies* intervenes in dominant presumptions of deservedness in relation to compassion. It shares a story of struggle with and survival from addiction and the glocal context of its assemblage.

While there are no explicit references to practices of addiction recovery usually spoken of within recovery communities, the culmination of the narrative gestures towards a movement away from the time-space of active addiction. This indicates that experiences of recovery do not all conform to established conventions. Lewis noted in his criticism of the predominance of the disease (medical) concept of addiction that 'addicts who end up quitting do so uniquely and inventively, through effort and insight' (2016, xiv). He proposed that instead of the term recovery, cessation of addiction activity should be framed as 'further development' (xiv). In the final section of *Like Butterflies*, Shelly demonstrates her further development in getting a job and setting goals for the future that involve a deeper insight into her interactions with others and herself. The monologue culminates with the image of Shelly, years later and having earned enough to buy her own van, driving off 'to sunsets, hills, valleys' (2018, 12) full of excitement about the potential future that lies ahead.

Ideas of place, as shown above, contribute to an enhanced understanding of assemblages of addiction and the non-normative spaces of dwelling in which addicted people inhabit. How might ideas of place, subsequently, inform a better understanding of how we might construct environments that nurture multiple and varied trajectories of recovery?

Recovery Attachments to Place

To celebrate the twentieth anniversary of Outside Edge Theatre Company, an Open House event was conceived and organised by the new Artistic Director, Matt Steinberg. Past and present participants, trustees, patrons, friends, staff, supporters and other local service users were invited to join to 'celebrate the company's history and help us plan the future of Outside Edge' on the evening of 2 November 2018.[6] The invitation stated that in the afternoon 'we are turning 61 Munster Road into the creative hub for south-west London, showcasing the incredible talent in our community'. Recipients were also invited to contribute a performance or food towards a potluck meal.

On the evening of the event I arrived at 61 Munster Road, a period property on an affluent residential road in south-west London converted into a community services facility. I was welcomed at the door by a new member of Outside Edge and provided with a sticky label to write my name on. Already inside were members of the board of trustees and one of the patrons, with whom I exchanged greetings. Others who had arrived early were already in the kitchen making themselves a cup of tea or coffee, as I know is the usual routine. The large room at the back of the house had a small stage above which were gold and silver balloons spelling OETC20. Throughout the evening Steinberg compered a wide selection of performances on themes relating to addiction and recovery from those who had responded to the call for participation. Performances included extracts from plays written and performed by people in recovery and also family members of those affected by addiction, a monologue set within a group therapy session, a provocative poem about recovery, a stand-up comedy act, a dance performance from Fallen Angels

Dance Theatre, a rendition of the song 'Tainted Love', and a sharing from former trustee and ongoing supporter David Charkham.

At the front of the building, two of the meeting rooms had been cleared, their doorways decorated with coloured lights and each had large sheets of paper on the walls. Written on these sheets were questions to provoke discussion on key themes such as the future of the company and the role of peer support. These spaces became the site for discussion and reflection later in the evening, when Steinberg invited audience members to break away from the large room during scheduled intervals between performances. Ideas were shared and recorded on the large pieces of paper.

The description above documents one of my many encounters with 61 Munster Road. This event, however, was particularly significant in that it marked my first return to Outside Edge's home base to view a performance since I had left the company in 2015. While not a literal home, given its conversion into a community treatment facility, 61 Munster Road had, for a time, felt like a homely place to me. During the Open House event, memories of old associations collided with new discoveries and hope for the future of the organisation and those connected to it. As Massey suggests, located space consists of a combination of 'stories-so-far' (the past) as well as 'multiple trajectories' (the present and future) (2005, 24). My discussion of 61 Munster Road in this chapter, therefore, provides a useful device with which to reveal how ideas of place can contribute to establishing situated 'atmospheres of recovery' (Duff 2016, 58).

An Alternative Homespace

Most of the activity of the Open House event occurred in a large room at the rear of the building. During the twenty years of Outside Edge's habitation of 61 Munster Road, this room facilitated workshops, rehearsals, meetings, celebrations and performance sharings. It was where, one evening in October 2011, that I met the founder of the company Phil Fox for the first time. I was a relatively new arrival to London, having just migrated from Northern Ireland to begin a Master's degree course in Applied Theatre. During this early period of excitement and of feeling overwhelmed in this strange city, 61 Munster Road became a place where I felt warmth and familiarity. I distinctly remember the circle of well-worn armchairs to the right-hand side of the door where I would sit on that first visit, and every subsequent visit, as company members would gather for the ritual check-in before every session. Strewn with slightly bobbled red felt throws and an assortment of cushions, the cosy, yet slightly tattered furniture evoked a sense of relaxed warmth that perhaps assisted the sense of welcome that participants would reflect upon when asked to describe their experience at Outside Edge. I also remember the paradoxical comfort the chair circle offered on the evening in June 2014 when I had the difficult task of sharing the unexpected news of Fox's sudden death to members of the company. After an extended check-in, we chose to play some of his favourite warm-up games because staying in this room, being together amid the familiar inhabitants of this space, felt comforting. Over the following weeks, several former participants returned to the scheduled workshop groups, showing a desire to spend time in this room, with fellow Outside Edgers.

Mackey and Whybrow warn of the limitations and 'misconceived idealism' of nostalgia regarding ideas of place in applied performance contexts (2007, 2). It is not, therefore, a nostalgic connection with 61 Munster Road that I share, but rather an acknowledgement of the way in which the experience of the performance practices of Outside Edge were enmeshed with the more-than-human surroundings. For instance, the electric hand dryer in the toilet adjacent to the workshop room would regularly interrupt proceedings with its high-pitched whirring. On occasion, if we had forgotten to switch it off beforehand, it would feature in a performance sharing when an audience member attempted to surreptitiously use the bathroom during the show. Such quirks, including the doorstop that would spontaneously release and slam the door shut, were nonhuman contributors to an environment in which imperfection was embraced. They were the distinctive features of the liminal homespace of Outside Edge.

Home, for people affected by addiction, is often complicated and messy. As Maté's discussion of his addicted patients suggests, neglect, abuse or trauma experienced at a very early age can produce neuro-psychological conditions that might lead to addiction in later life (2013, 154–156). It is important to note that experience of family abuse or neglect does not precipitate all experiences of addiction as there are many and varied factors influencing individual experience. Addiction is, however, often referred to as a 'family disease' (Roth 2010) in that it impacts those closest to the addicted person and patterns of co-dependency, estrangement and mental health difficulties within family networks are exacerbated by cycles of active addiction. Supporting the whole family is considered by some addiction treatment specialists as an essential part of addiction recovery (Lander et al. 2013, 204). People affected by addiction might also experience periods of itinerant life, be that through homelessness or through an active choice to 'do a geographic'.[7] The location of home might also be associated with experiences of wider societal oppressions such as racism and homophobia. Practitioners involved in recovery-engaged arts activity must, therefore, appreciate the complicatedness of ideas of home within recovery communities which might entail a desire for belonging contradicted by an ambivalence to located or past vestiges of home.

Drawing on Una Chaudhuri's discussion of theatre as a type of home, constructed through shared experience rather than ownership, Lisa Woynarski's ecodramaturgies offer an understanding of how performance practice can extend ideas of home through manifesting, amplifying and critiquing aspects of home and place (2020, 145).

At 61 Munster Road, the creative practices of Outside Edge contributed to a construction of place contingent upon the diverse bodies, human and nonhuman, interacting through recovery-engaged arts activity. The building did not belong to Outside Edge. Use of the premises was granted rent-free by the local authority in agreement with the successive charitable organisations that had won the tender for providing addiction support services in the building. There was always, therefore, a sense of precarity in that shared use of rooms within the building were frequently under negotiation and could be contested or restricted according to the priorities of the incumbent service's managers. Yet through the sharing of recovery experience and creative interaction with the nonhuman aspects of this site, a form of dwelling instigated a sense of belonging that might be considered a form of homeliness.

In previous writing, I applied Victor Turner's term 'communitas' (1982) to denote the feeling of belonging felt by company participants during collective performance-related activity (Sloan 2014, 228). I have since shifted my thinking to include an appreciation of space and the more-than-human in the creative encounter. It is still useful to note that participants interviewed for my initial research referred to participation at Outside Edge as feeling 'like a family' (228). I do not infer any idealistic idea of family here, but simply refer to the way in which participants reported feelings of inclusion, nonjudgemental validation and acceptance as well as experiences of guidance and mentorship in how to navigate social interactions within the group (299). The practices of Outside Edge, therefore, generated an atmosphere of recovery in which people in recovery might thrive. 'Becoming well', according to Duff, is best facilitated through 'the staging of atmospheres of recovery' that address the ways in which recovery is impacted by affects, spaces and bodies of any given assemblage of addiction (2016, 58). An affective atmosphere could be conducive to recovery in how it nurtures an increased capacity for sociability, enabling connections with people and place that might lead to a sense of belonging and also hope (67–69). Duff also highlighted the importance of duration, atmospheres that can be sustained in everyday practices and encounters (72).

Sustained connections and practices were evident at the Open House event with the presence of familiar faces and rituals, from tea-making in the communal kitchen to recovery-attuned chitchat on the metal bistro-style chairs in the small, paved garden. By the end of the evening's proceedings Steinberg had facilitated the sharing of a plethora of performances on the theme of addiction and he had also, I suggest, generated a *space of potentiality* through the affective experience of the social and performative interactions from which emerged new ideas and connections for the future development of the company. For example, the 'brainstorming' sessions had gathered ideas from those with past and/or present attachments to Outside Edge, inviting them to imagine how they might be involved in its future. The assemblage of people in shared participation (or spectating) reunited and generated connection with former participants, potential new members, new donors and possible partner organisations.

Transporting Place

The inception of the Open House event was, nonetheless, a reminder that place, as Mackey pointed out, is composed of temporary periods of dwelling (2016, 110). The layers of activity and interaction that occurred in the description I provided earlier were a creative response to the precarious circumstances of Outside Edge that Steinberg encountered when he became Artistic Director in June 2018. During a conversation with Steinberg in September 2018, he revealed that the financial security of the organisation was worsened by continued cuts to core funding from the local tri-borough substance misuse and offender care (SMOC) team and the conclusion of pre-existing short-term funding contracts, leaving a significant gap in income to support the work of the company. Most pressing was the imminent homelessness of the organisation in that Outside Edge's residency at Munster Road was under review given that the building required substantial renovation and its shared tenants at the time, Turning Point drug and alcohol support services, had subsequently relocated elsewhere. Hammersmith and Fulham council (formerly in collaboration with Kensington and Chelsea council until 2018) had intervened to allow Outside Edge to remain in the building for six months to allow time for a solution to be found. During these interim months, Outside Edge would be the sole occupants of the building, thus enabling Steinberg to organise an event whereby Outside Edge would use every room on the ground floor.

Reflecting back on the Open House in a recorded conversation with me in October 2021, Steinberg noted that the event was in part a 'celebration of that space [Munster Road]'. He shared that it had become clear to him during the first summer of his tenure as Artistic Director that the 'physical building was really central to a lot of people's identity, their recovery identity, but also their understanding of what Outside Edge was'. His intention was, therefore, to quickly develop an understanding of these attachments while also publicly celebrating and documenting this cultural asset to make a case for the local authority to support maintaining Outside Edge's presence there. Although Outside Edge was granted permission to remain in the building for longer than the initial six-month notice, it was eventually given final notice to quit at the beginning of 2020 because the council had at this point decided to 'redevelop' the property. Incidentally, Outside Edge's departure from the building coincided with the first UK lockdown in March 2020 in response to the COVID-19 pandemic. Steinberg reflected on his concerns about Outside Edge 'losing a sense of home', especially as this seemed important to participants

> because of that sense of protection. So many of them come from places where they don't really think they have homes anymore, or don't have a home that feels like theirs. I think that Outside Edge was able to establish that for twenty years, for some people. We still have some of the same service users coming to us ... from twenty years ago'
> (Personal conversation with the author in 2021)

At the time of the Open House event in November 2018, it was difficult for me to envision an Outside Edge separate from 61 Munster Road; however, I was very aware that this charitable organisation did not have the financial capacity to take on the expense of the rent and structural renovation required, although this option had initially been offered by the local authority. It was evident that Outside Edge would need to find a new base, preferably an agreed cohabitation within an existing arts venue or community hub. What would be the consequences of moving home, however? Fortunately, Steinberg's vision for the company stretched beyond a nostalgic attachment to what had gone before. As indicated earlier, Mackey and Whybrow highlight that nostalgic attachment to place can result in territorialisation and defensive boundary-making that leads to exclusion (2007, 6). In the context of Outside Edge, the impending end to its habitation at Munster Road provided an opportunity to reimagine its community membership beyond the geophysical sphere of south-west London and what the key practices and activities of the organisation could be, moving forward. The discussions held during the Open House event generated a space in which former and current members could participate in this reimagining.

Mackey suggests that, given the relational construction of place, it can be interpreted as 'provisional and transitional' (2016, 111). Challenging the binary of rootedness versus fluidity, she highlights how theatre practice can increase attachment to a new place or reimagine one's affinity to place (111). I extend these ideas of transitional place to consider if, perhaps, features of place might be transported to new locations. By this, I do not mean a literal moving of physical items, although moving to a different home does usually entail the movement of things. Rather, if space, as Massey proposes, is constructed through material practices that are 'always in the process of being made' (2005, 9), then perhaps the transportation of these practices to other sites might bring traces of the affective atmosphere of 61 Munster Road to new locations.

It is now summer in 2022, as I write this chapter, and the Open House event has since morphed into an annual RecoveryFest and barbeque. I receive an invitation to this year's gathering, recommencing the tradition after the hiatus imposed by social distancing regulations during the COVID-19 pandemic. Outside Edge's base is currently located within Brady Arts Centre in Whitechapel, east London. In October 2021, as lockdown measures were eased, I visited Steinberg at Brady Arts Centre. As I entered the building, it was apparent that the cohabitation arrangement enabled the local activities and administration of Outside Edge to be enmeshed in a more diverse, arts-based environment. Steinberg and I chatted in the café area, surrounded by a mix of young and older members of the community. Moving to the large hall, we perched on the edge of the stage to conduct the recorded conversation for this research, pausing occasionally as other community facilitators popped in to retrieve items from the store cupboard. There was a convivial atmosphere. It was heartening for me to witness the transportation of Outside Edge's creative practices of dwelling beyond the location of addiction treatment buildings. This achievement is particularly of note in its potential to shift stereotypes of people affected by addiction as the 'dangerous other' (Lorey 2015, 38).

Extending Butler's ideas on cohabitation to the dwelling of Outside Edge, I observe the potential of its contribution to co-construct spaces and places in wider community in which 'a liveable interdependency becomes possible' (2015, 69). I do not suggest an idealistic or co-dependent interpretation of interdependency here, but rather, as Butler suggests, I acknowledge that 'everyone is precarious' and vulnerable to political and social structures that can impact on survival (118). Recovery-engaged arts practices not only reveal that life – a form of being – beyond addiction is possible, but can also demonstrate how recovery communities can coexist among the wider society and disrupt the flawed dichotomy of them and us, deviant and productive citizen.

In contrast to Outside Edge's previous attachment to one location, Steinberg has developed a series of satellite groups that operate in sites across London. Drop-in drama workshops and script writing groups are currently facilitated in community venues in South and West London in addition to the company base in the East. All groups currently have blended delivery, incorporating online access and there is a regular peer-led check-in group hosted online every Friday. Outside Edge now reaches more participants across London than it did while located at the fixed address of 61 Munster Road. It is also involved in performance collaborations with other leading UK recovery arts organisations, such as the Moving Recovery project with Fallen Angels Dance Theatre which is based in Manchester and the Overdose Awareness Day initiative led by Brighton-based Small Performance Adventures.

This growth emerged despite, and perhaps was aided by, the events of the global pandemic that impacted the organisation in 2020–2021. In the weeks preceding the first UK national lockdown in March 2020, Steinberg and project administrator, Molly Cox, sought practical solutions to the new dilemmas they were then encountering as Outside Edge entered a phase of remote delivery whereby activities would be facilitated at workshop spaces within community venues across London while a more permanent base was found. The administrative hub would, until further notice, be separate from the creative workshop locations. Steinberg was concerned about how to mutate the existing, settled practices of the company to a distanced model, while still ensuring safeguarding and appropriate support for participants and facilitators. Following the imposition of a national lockdown and, subsequently, the enforcement of social distancing measures that remained in place until July 2021, Steinberg found an ironic sense of relief in that the 'whole world' was now grappling with similar problems of how to supervise remote delivery and develop digital infrastructures for activities that had previously been bound to a geophysical place.

With the emergence of free access to video conferencing platforms such as Zoom and the mass turn towards digital communication as a surrogate for the now prohibited in-person contact, Steinberg found that they were rapidly able to meet their goals for the wider reach and digital distribution of Outside Edge's work. Facilitators quickly redesigned their activities to incorporate the newly available technology and most participants embraced this new way of being as a mode of resilience to the global crises with which they were surrounded. There were, nonetheless, challenges in assisting some with access to digital technology and providing guidance in how to use unfamiliar methods of communication. In the early stages of the first lockdown, Outside Edge focused on maintaining connection through any means possible, including text messages, to provide wellbeing support. Steinberg recalled how they shifted the organisation's immediate funding strategy to obtain the means to provide digital tablets and data cards to participants as a form of welfare support. He estimated that, unfortunately, they lost contact with approximately one-third of all the participants who had been attending workshops before the lockdown. Conversely, there was an additional number of people that had not engaged for years, but suddenly returned through engaging with the online services. The peer-led Friday support group was initially instigated by the participants and continues to be organised by them, demonstrating the collective action of community that was able to engage and exist beyond a fixed location of Outside Edge.

As illustrated above, through creative practices, Outside Edge was able to shift geophysical attachments and transport the recovery-engaged atmosphere of the company to other sites, including the virtual. Nonetheless, the swift return to in-person delivery and collective gatherings reinforced the fact that the live, located experience of place still matters.

Conclusion

The examples of *Like Butterflies* and the Open House event, discussed in this chapter, reveal the importance of place in understanding contextualised experiences of addiction and recovery. Both reveal forms of dwelling that challenge stereotypes based on hierarchies of social value and imposition of hegemonic norms.

The cohabitations of Outside Edge, in particular, illustrate how recovery-engaged arts practice can generate atmospheres of recovery that might even offer alternative temporary homespaces for people for whom quotidian connotations of home are messy and problematic. The transportation of atmospheres of recovery is made possible through attachments to the recovery community, past and present.

Notes

1 The quotations from the solo play included in this chapter originate from a private copy of the rehearsal script that was sent to me by the author for research purposes. While the text is not publicly available, the author is happy to provide access to the unpublished text on request.

2 Cited from an interview with Sonya Hale to promote the staged production of her monologue *Dean McBride* which won the Heretic Productions writing competition and was performed at Arcola Theatre in January 2018. The interview was posted on Arcola Theatre's Facebook page, although is no longer available (accessed 25 May 2018).
3 'Council estate' is the term used in the UK for an area of public housing built by the local council authority.
4 I use the word 'grafting' here to indicate the broad spectrum of activities, including crime, that drug users may employ to acquire enough money to buy illicit substances. The reference to crime also challenges normative assumptions of morality. For instance, Shelly and T prefer to 'work' for money – work being shoplifting or other petty theft – rather than beg for money.
5 I include in my definition of women any person who identifies as feminine in gender.
6 Quoted from the invitation sent via email to all the company's contacts and circulated via social media.
7 'Doing a geographic' is a phrase used in recovery circles referring to the choice made during active addiction to move location, changing city or even country, with the expectation that this will interrupt the cycle of addiction and enable recovery.

References

Ahmed, S. (2010) 'Happy objects', in M. Gregg and G.J. Seigworth (eds), *The affect theory reader*. Durham, NC: Duke University Press, pp. 29–50.

Bennett, J. (2010) *Vibrant matter: A political ecology of things*. Durham, NC: Duke University Press.

Beswick, K. (2011) 'The council estate: Representation, space and the potential for performance', *Research in Drama Education: The Journal of Applied Theatre and Performance*, 16 (3), pp. 421–435. Available at: https://doi.org/10.1080/13569783.2011.589999.

Butler, J. (2015) *Notes toward a performative theory of assembly*. Cambridge, MA: Harvard University Press.

Campbell, N. and Ettorre, E. (2014) *Gendering addiction*. Basingstoke and New York: Palgrave Macmillan.

Downes, J. (2018) 'Sexual violence may be in the Hollywood spotlight, but there are limits to speaking out', *The Conversation*, 3 February. Available at: https://theconversation.com/sexual-violence-may-be-in-the-hollywood-spotlight-but-there-are-limits-to-speaking-out-92090 (accessed 6 May 2018).

Duff, C. (2014) *Assemblages of health: Deleuze's empiricism and the ethology of life*. New York: Springer.

Duff, C. (2016) 'Atmospheres of recovery: Assemblages of health', *Environment and Planning A*, 48 (1), pp. 58–74. Available at: https://doi.org/10.1177/0308518X15603222.

Edwards, E. (2018) *The political history of smack and crack*. London: Nick Hern Books.

Ettorre, E. (2015) 'Embodied deviance, gender, and epistemologies of ignorance: Re-visioning drugs use in a neurochemical, unjust world', *Substance Use & Misuse*, 50 (6), pp. 794–805. Available at: https://doi.org/10.3109/10826084.2015.978649.

Fisher, T. (2017) 'Introduction: Performance and the Tragic Politics of the Agōn', in T. Fisher and E. Katsouraki (eds), *Performing antagonism: Theatre, performance and radical democracy*. London: Palgrave Macmillan, pp. 1–20.

Freebody, K. and Finneran, M. (2021) *Critical themes in drama: Social, cultural and political analysis*. London: Routledge.

Halberstam, J. (2005) *In a queer time and place: Transgender bodies, subcultural lives*. New York: New York University Press.

Lander, L., Howsare, J. and Byrne, M. (2013) 'The impact of substance use disorders on families and children: From theory to practice', *Social Work in Public Health*, 28 (3–4), pp. 194–205. Available at: https://doi.org/10.1080/19371918.2013.759005.

Lewis, M.D. (2016) *The biology of desire: Why addiction is not a disease*. Melbourne and London: Scribe Publications.

Lorey, I. (2015) *State of insecurity: Government of the precarious*. A. Derieg (trans.). London and New York: Verso.

Mackey, S. (2016) 'Performing location: Place and applied theatre', in J. Hughes and H. Nicholson (eds), *Critical perspectives on applied theatre*. Cambridge and New York: Cambridge University Press, pp. 107–122.

Mackey, S. and Whybrow, N. (2007) 'Taking place: Some reflections on site, performance and community', *Research in Drama Education: The Journal of Applied Theatre and Performance*, 12 (1), pp. 1–14. Available at: https://doi.org/10.1080/13569780601094785.

Manning, E. (2007) *Politics of touch: Sense, movement, sovereignty*. Minneapolis: University of Minnesota Press.

Manning, E. (2013) *Always more than one: Individuation's dance*. Durham, NC: Duke University Press.

Massey, D.B. (2005) *For space*. London and Thousand Oaks, CA: SAGE.

Maté, G. (2013) *In the realm of hungry ghosts: Close encounters with addiction*. Mississauga, ON and London: Vintage Canada.

Mouffe, C. (2013) *Agonistics: Thinking the world politically*. London and New York: Verso.

Ong, A. (2018) 'The limits of access: The messy temporalities of hope and the negotiation of place', *Research in Drama Education: The Journal of Applied Theatre and Performance*, 23 (3), pp. 467–478. Available at: https://doi.org/10.1080/13569783.2018.1468242.

Pedwell, C. (2014) *Affective relations: The transnational politics of empathy*. New York: Palgrave Macmillan.

Roth, J.D. (2010) 'Addiction as a family disease', *Journal of Groups in Addiction & Recovery*, 5 (1), pp. 1–3. Available at: https://doi.org/10.1080/15560350903547189.

Sloan, C. (2014) 'From "Substance Misuse: The Musical" to "Double Whammy": The affect of Outside Edge Theatre Company', in J. Reynolds and Z. Zontou (eds), *Addiction and performance*. Newcastle upon Tyne: Cambridge Scholars Publishing, pp. 214–233.

UK Government (2022) Swift, Certain, Tough: New consequences for drug possession. London: HMSO. Available at:https://www.gov.uk/government/consultations/swift-certain-tough-new-consequences-for-drug-possession-white-paper/swift-certain-tough-new-consequences-for-drug-possession-accessible-version#:~:text=Consequences%20should%20be%20tough%2C%20but,receive%20a%20tier%203%20intervention.

Turner, V.W. (1982) *From ritual to theatre: The human seriousness of play*. New York: Performing Arts Journal Publications.

Woynarski, L. (2020) *Ecodramaturgies: Theatre, performance and climate change*. Cham: Palgrave Macmillan.

5 Sustaining Recovery Connections through Creative Kinship

Focusing on two projects initiated by Small Performance Adventures, Terminal Uniqueness and Overdose Awareness Day, this chapter highlights how relations of care were extended through recovery-engaged creative projects during the COVID-19 pandemic crisis of 2020–2021. Ideas of care in applied theatre are extended to offer insight into a recovery-orientated concept of 'care-full' practice.

The premise of this book, so far, highlights how interactions with people, places and things are crucial elements of how both assemblages of addiction and atmospheres of recovery are constructed. As stated in the Introduction, recovery involves growing less harmful connections with people, oneself, objects and place. Ongoing practices of recovery, therefore, require ongoing interactions with environments conducive to recovery and, for many, this translates as connection with recovery communities. Connection with others is, inherently, 'messy' as we navigate the affective, emotive and indeterminate elements of any encounter. Recovery-engaged arts practice can assist with the development of new social networks and strengthen interpersonal skills (Kewley 2019, 2). Given the precarity of recovery itself and its dependency on ongoing connection to forms of recovery community, arts projects in this field should be viewed in terms of their involvement in crafting long-term relations of care that recognise interdependency as a strength as well as encourage the development of the participant's independence. This is, however, complicated, by existing funding models that focus on short term, stand-alone projects.

In this chapter, I attend to examples of how recovery-engaged arts have sustained caring connections with participants and operated as a creative recovery community. Specifically, I draw on two projects initiated by Small Performance Adventures' Artistic Director, Kate McCoy, namely Terminal Uniqueness and Overdose Awareness Day. Both projects illustrate how collaborative arts activity can generate recovery-attuned connections within and across arts organisations, with capacity for global reach through digital technology. Objects and place also feature as collaborators in the arts activities discussed below. These projects, pertinently, highlight efforts to sustain caring relations with others despite the obstacles of lockdown, social distancing and travel restrictions imposed during the COVID-19 pandemic.

DOI: 10.4324/9781003271062-6

Recovery Society

In March 2020, as the global spread of COVID-19 and an increase in the number of infections had precipitated the announcement of the first UK national lockdown, I received an invitation to join a Facebook group called Terminal Uniqueness. I quickly recognised the source of the invitation, from Small Performance Adventures, a participatory arts organisation based in Brighton, UK, which devises performances and facilitates workshops with people 'affected by life'.[1] On accepting the invitation, I joined a virtual community of performers, artists, musicians, arts practitioners and participants who had in common a shared understanding of the potential for creative activity to support and nurture wellbeing. Some had lived experience of recovery from addiction and/or mental health issues. Some were arts professionals who facilitate practice with people in recovery. The distinction between practitioner and participant was, however, intentionally blurred. After all, we were entering this unfamiliar era of lockdown life together through which we would all be experiencing a range of difficulties and trepidation.

In conversation with me in December 2020, McCoy explained that the name of the project, Terminal Uniqueness, was inspired by her discovery of its use within addiction recovery communities, particularly in the USA, to denote a version of 'personal exceptionalism'. Many US-based addiction service websites offer a definition of this term for their service users and the following quote from the Recovery Village provides a useful explanation of its relevance to addiction recovery.

> Terminal uniqueness is a way of thinking that can interfere with successful recovery and lead to relapse and overdose, which may be fatal. The condition allows people to defy facts and rationalize their behaviors because they believe their case is special.[2]

Prior to the outbreak of the pandemic, McCoy's original aim for the Terminal Uniqueness project was to explore how creative workshops, led by artists-in-recovery, might help to improve mental health collectively and so challenge individualism regarding mental wellbeing recovery. Small Performance Adventures would be assisted by Edit Sweet, a recovery filmmaking company, and We Are Not Saints, a music label founded by and for music artists-in-recovery. All three organisations are based in Brighton and frequently collaborate. McCoy light-heartedly referred to this blended collaboration as 'the small sweet saints'. By the spring of 2020, six artists had been commissioned and each had identified the community identity groups with which they wished to work. The first workshops were scheduled for 19 March 2020, but were cancelled as news of the spread of COVID-19 in the UK and the government's announcement of an imminent lockdown indicated that there might be a serious health risk for participants, one of whom was over eighty years old, should the planned workshops continue. After an emergency meeting with the respective artistic directors of the 'small sweet saints', the decision was made to go online. This began as a Facebook group with the simple instruction to members to share pictures or short videos of objects in their home on the theme of a given colour. They were inundated with contributions from a membership that quickly grew to over 800 members from across the globe, including Nigeria, Namibia, the Philippines, the USA and several cities in the UK. As use of digital conferencing became more prevalent, McCoy embraced access to Zoom to meet with her creative team and to plan artistic commissions whereby artists-in-recovery from within the group would create artworks in response to material from the Facebook posts. This culminated in a series of films that were edited by Edit Sweet and streamed live during watch parties hosted on the Terminal Uniqueness Facebook page in November 2020.

The Terminal Uniqueness project highlights the desire for connection during difficult times. This temporary virtual community facilitated online interaction that reminded its members that they were not alone and that sharing experiences, even simply a story about an everyday item in our home, can support collective wellbeing. This gathering of people created a recovery community of sorts, or perhaps what might aptly be called a survival community given the context. My use of the term community here appreciates the very particular connotations of this word within what Mark Prest, founder of Portraits of Recovery, has referred to as 'an emergent marginalised community' that, according to Prest, has been recognised by treatment services in the UK since 2010 (2018). Recovery communities have, however, existed long prior to this. For instance, the global networks of the Twelve Steps movement which emerged from the first Alcoholics Anonymous (AA) fellowship founded by Bill W. and Dr Bob S. in Akron, Ohio, 1935, might well be considered as a covert recovery community (Alcoholics Anonymous 1997). Bound by a pledge of anonymity, those following the Twelve Steps programme connect with a community held together through modes of peer support and relation to shared experience. The recent recognition that Prest refers to is, perhaps, due to the move in public health policy to recognise the effectiveness of the Twelve Steps programme to assist prolonged cycles of recovery, underpinned by research over the past decade indicating the increased likelihood of sustained abstinence when engaged with peer support groups (Tracy and Wallace 2016, 144).

There have also been moves from within the covert community of recovery to reach outwards. This is noticeable through the actions of individuals such as Russell Brand, who has made use of his celebrity to raise awareness of the insights of recovery from addiction,[3] and from the approval by the UK AA congress in 2018 of public posters with QR codes that, when scanned by a mobile phone would provide details of local meetings.[4] There is even, currently, an All Party Parliamentary Group for the Twelve Steps, established in March 2020, to make policy recommendations to the UK government on the role of Twelve Steps recovery in addiction treatment. New organisations have also emerged, such as the Scottish Recovery Consortium and Faces & Voices of Recovery (FAVOR) UK which hold public events to make visible recovery communities as well as to advocate for 'policy reform on issues of discrimination, social justice and access to recovery services'.[5] Both groups are involved in the organisation of the now annual Recovery Walks held in Scotland, England and Wales, respectively. These take the form of carnivalesque parades, not unlike the Pride marches of the LGBTQ+ community, during which people in recovery, their families and those involved in recovery services join together to celebrate and promote that recovery is possible.

In addition to understanding the specific features of recovery communities, I acknowledge the connotations of the term 'community' with regard to applied theatre practice, whereby there is an appreciation of it as a 'loaded term' that can mythologise idealised ideas of community cohesion through the arts (Freebody and Finneran 2021, 85). Applied performances often occur within community contexts and can represent and reinvent community identities. Community membership can, however, become associated with boundary-setting and exclusion. McAvinchey also highlights the limitations of groups formed around a specific issue or identity as 'being something', such as homeless or prisoner, and, consequently neglecting the 'glorious complexity of human beings' and the fluid, contradictory nature of identities (2014, 6). Applying the tenets of recovery community within recovery-engaged arts practice can, perhaps, ameliorate these limitations in that membership is on the basis of self-identification. Community, therefore, becomes a loose, fluid alliance of those who identify as being-in-recovery.

Practitioners in the field of recovery-engaged arts work with an awareness of lives 'in process' beyond active addiction and painful experience. There is a sense of identities in flux as participants grow in their recovery practices and adopt new ways of being in relation to their surroundings. Such arts practice, through its incorporation of people in recovery, connects with a multifaceted community that spans beyond any one geographical location and across the intersections of society. Perhaps then, it might be pertinent to adopt Ridout's proposal to substitute the word 'community' for 'society' when considering the communitarian potential of theatre (2013, 137). To quote his words, society more aptly infers 'a changeable association made of multiple conversations, across the intimate distances of the public space, rather than as a community that might close around its participants' (137). In this broader-reaching sense, the Terminal Uniqueness project demonstrates an approach to community that reaches beyond the local activity of any one organisation towards the national and global dimensions of recovery society.

By connecting individuals from across the globe through arts activities, the recovery-engaged practice of the 'small sweet saints' generated a temporary kinship that was supportive to wellbeing during a time of fear and social isolation. Even when my own struggle with long COVID inhibited me from actively contributing to the group after its initial launch, viewing the activities via the Facebook posts and streamed films still provided me with a vicarious attachment to this community that enabled me to feel connected to a recovery-orientated network beyond the confines of my home.

Manning's concept of 'life-living' is particularly relevant in how it offers an ethos of lived existence as composed by interconnections and, importantly, interdependency (2016, p.8). As discussed throughout this book, recovery from addiction involves a complex assemblage of contributing factors that extend beyond the individual. The COVID-19 pandemic has also reminded us of our collective responsibilities to prevent harm to others by doing what we can to inhibit the spread of a virus that, for many, can be a mild illness but that can be fatal for the elderly and vulnerable people. An ethos of 'life-living', enabled by arts practices such as Small Performance Adventures' project discussed above, might therefore offer an antidote to the individualist malaise of *terminal uniqueness*.

'Making Kin' in Troubled Times

Performance projects, by their collaborative nature, enable modes of connection and a sense of community which might be conceived as a form of kinship. The kinship to which I refer is not that of biological ancestry or even conventional family attachments; rather, drawing on queer kinship theory, it imagines a 'belonging otherwise' (Bradway and Freeman 2022, 2). While queer kinship denotes specific lineages and attachments through sexual identity, the emphasis on 'relationality' and 'sodality' (2) translates aptly to the ways in which a recovery community operates. As mentioned in the previous chapter, associations of home and family kinship can be painful and difficult for those impacted by active addiction. Alternative modes of kinship-in-recovery might then offer modes of sociability that support a moving beyond addiction. In particular, Bradway and Freeman's concept of kin-aesthetics highlights how belonging is enacted through social practices or imaginative texts that de-form and re-form the social field (4). Practices of recovery and, in the context of this book, recovery-engaged artistic practices, form, re-form and reimagine the social contexts of people-in-recovery. The communal and interdependent elements of these practices, particularly in the rituals of Twelve Steps recovery group meetings and sponsorship, convey lineages of recovery knowledge and practice.

The arts organisations involved in the field of addiction recovery arts practice, such as Small Performance Adventures, have simultaneous attachments to recovery-engaged modes of practice, recovery community and also tangentially to each other and to past and future legacies amid the field of recovery-engaged arts. Knowledges of recovery and recovery-engaged performance practice are transmitted through interactions that operate as a form of archive-repertoire. As Diana Taylor asserts in *The Archive and the Repertoire* (2003), an archive need not be a written or static documentation of the past (19). Taylor aptly addressed the role of performance research in attending to embodied expression as participating in the 'transmission of knowledge, memory, and identity pre- and post-writing' (16). So too do the examples discussed in this book transfuse embodied ways of knowing and ways of creating, that, as Taylor noted, require 'presence' and 'participation' (20). Taylor's emphasis on the postcolonial project of privileging the affective mean-making of the social scenario in relation to its milieu is relevant to my own attempt in this book to capture the affective relations of practices and people that would not be recognised in traditional performance canons.

Small Performance Adventures' iterative Overdose Awareness Day (OAD) project has initiated creative collaborations with several recovery arts organisations across the UK. In doing so, it represents an example of not only connections across a national recovery arts community, but also shares an ethos of recovery-engaged practice between organisations. Beginning in the summer of 2020, McCoy led a series of creative sessions via Zoom in which selected performers from each of the participating organisations explored physical gestures that were to form the movement sequences for the OAD performance. Initially, as with the Terminal Uniqueness project discussed above, the OAD project was intended to be a live performance. McCoy's original concept was that arts organisations around the UK specialising in addiction recovery would simultaneously perform a series of short pop-up movement sequences in local public spaces to draw attention to the annual commemoration of International Overdose Awareness Day.

Initiated in 2001 by Sally Finn in Melbourne, Australia, International Overdose Awareness Day occurs on the 31 August every year. Activities co-ordinated by the Australian public health organisation, Pennington Institute, aim to encourage awareness of deaths by drug- and alcohol-related harm, remember those who have died, honour the grief felt by loved ones and advocate for better approaches to overdose prevention. Overall, it seeks to disrupt the stigma around deaths caused by addiction that further exacerbates the pain of loss felt by those impacted by it and those still struggling with substance dependencies. Small Performance Adventures' project intersects with this international movement, seeking to raise awareness of the increasing number of deaths by drug- and alcohol-related overdose in the UK. For instance, Release, the drug awareness charity, issued a press release in 2021 that highlighted the continued increase in the number of deaths by drug poisoning; there were 4,561 deaths in England and Wales in 2020 which constituted the highest number since records began in 1993. Small Performance Adventures' project indicates its 'recoverist' activism, in that it endeavours to reveal and represent lived experiences of recovery with the intention of social justice for those marginalised by the stigma of substance addiction.

The *Recoverist Manifesto* positioned recovery as a civil rights issue (Parkinson, 2015). Launched in 2015 as an output of a European Union-funded arts project with people in recovery from addiction,[6] the manifesto represented opinions expressed by participants about 'the frustration of everyday lived experience and the assumptions and myths that surround addiction' (3). It concluded with a poem that pledged a commitment to solidarity and a demand for equality (8). Thus, the term 'recoverist' denotes a political act of commitment to making visible the perspectives and struggles of people in recovery. In short, a recoverist is considered a recovery activist.

The onset of the COVID-19 pandemic disrupted McCoy's initial plans for live pop-up performances across England, with social distancing measures rendering collaborative rehearsals, travel and public performance difficult. Determined to continue with the project, McCoy, assisted by film company Edit Sweet, reinterpreted the creative concept to take advantage of the upsurge in engagement with online and digital technology at the time. The project became a curated film, capturing devised movement sequences in outdoor spaces where participating arts organisations were located. These locations included Brighton, London, Plymouth and Bristol. Only the filmmaker would travel to each group, complying to the respective region's social distancing measures at the time. Zoom sessions served as a substitute for in-person rehearsals combining all organisations to devise a thematic gesture that would feature in the varied iterations of the filmed movement sequences. McCoy, reflecting on feedback from participants after the 2020 project cycle, noted the positive response to meeting and collaborating online (personal conversation with the author). She admitted that had it not been for the pandemic, they would not have used digital technology to connect the collaborators in joint session, in which case they would have probably worked in isolation in their respective locations. Ironically, the pandemic had precipitated closer collaboration and interaction than perhaps would have occurred.

When viewing the finished film that was streamed on social media on 30 August 2020, it was evident that the nonhuman geographical features of outdoor environments were key contributors to the performance. For instance, in the sequence captured on the beachfront in Brighton, the sea is a powerful performer. The repetitive lapping of waves against the human performers' bodies and a lone stargazer lily floating out to the horizon evoke compelling references to time, attrition and loss. Additionally, the graffiti-ridden concrete walls in an underground passageway shot in Plymouth impose on the solitary human performer a sombre gravity. In Bristol, trees frame the scene in which a stretch of grass catches fallen human bodies. The enduring vegetation denote a contrast to the transitory movements of the human. Without the nonhuman elements of the filmed sequences, the *affect* of the overall performance would be significantly lessened. They assist in conveying the gesture of remembrance and grief that was the overall aim of the project. Small Performance Adventures' subsequent OAD performance in August 2021 further incorporated nonhuman topography with drone footage capturing the panoramic environmental context of the miniaturised human performers. This time Birmingham, Chester and Manchester were added to the previous list of locations.

Donna Haraway's posthuman approach to kinship highlights the need for an affinity with other 'earthly critters', reminding us that subjective human experience is entangled with our nonhuman cohabitors (2016, 2). In *Staying with the Trouble*, kinship in the present moment is set within a chthulucene[7] marked as 'disturbing' and 'turbid' times, containing a 'damaged earth' (2). Making kin, in Haraway's sense, therefore requires 'inventive connection' with the nonhuman as a practice of learning to 'live and die well with each other in a thick present' (1). People-in-recovery, with their attunement to pain and survival, know this all too well. My discussions of recovery and recovery-engaged performance practice throughout this book highlight the nonhuman contributors to human experiences of addiction and recovery. It follows, therefore, that the collaborative artistry of Small Performance Adventures' OAD project demonstrates the ways in which recovery-engaged approaches to performance encompass the material surroundings in which people-in-recovery are enmeshed. Likewise, the Terminal Uniqueness initiative hinged on the performative gestures of images and videos of objects whose colour, shape and form generated and inspired the artistic content.

Perpetual Recovery and Sustained Relations of Care

Given my emphasis on the theme of survival in this book, it is important to return to the precarity of recovery and reflect on how the recovery-engaged arts practices discussed in this chapter relate to this process. Drawing on Manning's concept of 'life-living' mentioned earlier (2016, 3–8), I propose here that by acknowledging interdependency as a feature of all life, including the more-than-human, such arts practices are better conceived as a nexus for recovery society rather than temporary short-term projects. By this, I suggest that they might operate as localised creative hubs, simultaneously embedded in and facilitating connection to forms of recovery community.

As identified in Chapter 1, I consider recovery from addiction as a practice of survival which involves commitment to developing new ways of being-in-the-world that enable someone to move beyond the overwhelming cycle of active addiction. At its core, recovery-engaged arts practices might be considered as emerging from acts of survival from addiction and are concerned with supporting ongoing recovery. For instance, Phil Fox stated that his 'addict life was based on survival' (2014, 359). Indeed, processes of survival marked Fox's life in very particular ways: survival from childhood abuse; survival from mental illness; survival from traumatic experiences incurred during active addiction; and, ultimately, survival from heroin addiction (359–365). By the time Fox reached his late twenties, he had exchanged drug use for a new and more constructive process of survival which was theatre-making and the eventual creation of Outside Edge Theatre Company. The narratives of the many plays he subsequently wrote or devised and directed also entailed narratives of survival from the experiences of people affected by addiction.[8] Fox attributed his recovery to the impact of his involvement with theatre-making (366). Moreover, several of the artists involved in the practices discussed throughout this book would attribute their arts practice as part of their ongoing recovery process.

If recovery is a long-term and gradual process of developing strategies for resilience that enables regeneration, and relapse a potential part of the recovery experience, then any provision of recovery support must acknowledge the criticality of networks and cycles of connection to modes of peer support. Long-term engagement with practices of recovery recognises that collective interdependency is a strength and is necessary for survival. The neoliberal concept of self-care places responsibility on the individual to sustain themselves as effective citizens. Yet, in offering the concept of co-habitation, Butler has highlighted our 'reciprocal obligations' to each other (2015, 218). Those in recovery, I suggest, are already aware of the necessity of connection for regeneration and in surrounding oneself with connections that will inform and support their chosen recovery practice.

Hence, Manning's discussion of 'life-living' (2016, 8) as a way of living life that is more-than-human equates with the philosophical conception of the experience of *being in recovery* that I propose in this book. Responding to issues relating to disability rights campaigns and the #BlackLivesMatter global network, she proposed life-living as a turn away from the values imposed by tenets of neurotypicality that reinforce white western-centric hegemonic norms in the global north (2016, 3). Life-living, therefore, entails not only recognising but honouring how complex forms of interdependency are a feature of life and how we might create encounters that embrace difference (5).

I suggest that recovery-engaged arts projects that instigate encounters of recovery community operate as a *minor gesture* (Manning 2016) towards acknowledging the contingency of life in recovery as a collective and interdependent process. It is imperative, therefore, to consider how practitioners and organisations might sustain their attachments to the collectives of people in recovery that emerge. This raises the concern of sustainability of practice that has been discussed at length in applied theatre literature. To maintain attachments to the localised recovery arts communities that emerge from arts projects and organisations, it is important to adopt a long-term approach. As Busby indicated, the 'ripple of affect' towards change instigated by an applied theatre project may well be made possible because of its longevity (2017, 102). Indeed, Thompson proposed an 'aesthetics of care' for applied theatre practice that emerges from relational processes between individuals and groups over time that could be realised in 'more enduring, crafted encounters between people' informed by mutual regard (2015, 437). Such extenuating attachments of care are similarly visible in the collaborations and iterative projects of the coalition of 'small sweet saints' discussed earlier. So too is my own research infused with relations of care with practitioners, performers and peers as we belong to a growing network of addiction-recovery arts practice.

Concurrently, I propose that recovery-engaged arts practice is not only bound and constituted by its attachments with recovery communities, but that modes of funding and organisational structure must address the need for long-term engagement with the members of recovery communities who seek to participate for an extended period of time. I note, however, that such attachments are not envisaged as modes of co-dependency that would infer entrapment and manipulation by the organisation, or well-meaning practitioner. Rather, as Thompson proposed, it is a 'dynamic system of relations' of care, imbued by 'invitation, dialogue and reciprocity', that serve as a counterpoint to the cruel disregard of contemporary society (439–440).

Investing in Community-Situated Creative Recovery

An emphasis on generating long-term attachments to a recovery community might, consequently, be a more efficacious approach to accounting for the potential impact of recovery-engaged arts practices. Developments generated by the work of researchers and practitioners advocating arts for and in health and the increased emphasis on community support for mental wellbeing offer potential new collaborative relationships. These developments also offer an opportunity to consider, or perhaps reimagine, how recovery-engaged arts practices survive economic precarity through their inclusion in new models of funding. Daisy Fancourt's research in the field of psychobiology has advocated for community engagement in arts and cultural activity as an additional mechanism for supporting recovery from illness in the broader context of health and wellbeing (2017). She highlighted the development of new commissioning models to include arts activity within the NHS in the UK, such as 'social prescribing' by which arts and culture are directly commissioned through the health budget (60). The movement towards what has been referred to as 'arts on prescription' in the media, was indicated by the production of a new health resource published by Health Education England entitled *Social Prescribing at a Glance* (2016).

The commissioning of arts activities as an adjunct to mental health services within communities has been documented as in existence since the 1990s, with public health researchers Bungay and Clift citing an early example in Stockport in 1994 (2010, 277). The report of the All Party Parliamentary Group (APPG) on arts, health and wellbeing published in 2017, however, raised the profile and urgency of making more effective use of the positive contribution of arts to recovery and wellbeing 'across the human life cycle, from the very young to the aging members of the population' (4). This corresponded with the launch of the Cultural Health and Wellbeing Alliance and London Arts in Health Forum in 2018. Post-pandemic, as communities emerge from prolonged social isolation, the rebuilding of social networks and in-person connections with recovery peers is ever more vital.

There is, perhaps, a risk that the emphasis on the purposefulness and quantifiable impact of arts in/for health as reflected in the reports published by Fancourt and the APPG leans towards the instrumentalisation of practices, an issue that has long been critiqued within the field of applied theatre. Veronica Baxter and Katherine Low have warned against 'medicalising the arts' (2017, 5) highlighting that while arts practice has great potential for positive impact on wellbeing, it should not be used as a '"salve" for widespread and complex social ills' (7). Emma Brodzinski emphasised the importance of practitioners maintaining focus on and communicating the aesthetic artistry of their work (2010, 16). In recognition of the difficulty of communicating imperatives and evaluation of practice across contrasting disciplines, Brodzinski offered the concept of 'the arts in health broker' who might act as a translator within the process (13). Like other language translators, this broker would have significant 'fluency' in the languages of the arts and health disciplines in order to facilitate shared agreement on 'realistic objectives' and ensure equal status of each discipline (13 and 15.) While such systems of brokerage seemed to have developed through the arts in health movement, addiction-recovery practices require an understanding of how they uniquely operate within and across recovery communities.

The continued growth and development of this field of practice is allied to how long-term connections might be embedded in situated recovery communities. Simultaneously, future events or collective encounters, such as Terminal Uniqueness and OAD discussed above, hold the potential to reach outwards in a 'minor gesture' towards a wider network of recovery society. In moving forward, such a network might offer a brokerage of funding processes and knowledge exchange that better supports the survival of the unique and vital practices of recovery-engaged arts. The relations of care and recovery-engaged perspectives that operate within these collectives offer forms of cohabitation that indicate a reimagining of a more inclusive democracy may emerge from the potential of such collaborative encounters.

Furthermore, as core treatment services have experienced cuts in funding, there is subsequently less funding available for arts projects that might be considered a value-added option, rather than an essential part of the programme. When faced with cuts to state funding, arts companies in this field can and do apply to private trust funds for financial support. These forms of funding tend to emphasise social impact criteria in their application processes. As McAvinchey has highlighted, this places an onus on the artist to articulate a particular promise in the framing of their practice (2014, 6). Such promises are antithetical to the reality of the artistry involved which, as Thompson argued, relies on the less easily communicated, and at times accidental, affects of a performance project (2011, 6). This is certainly relevant to art practice with recovery experiences that are vulnerable to relapse and that often entail a personal journey that involves renegotiating one's relation to the world. Long-term practices of recovery are not best facilitated through the imposition of social norms of what might be considered an effective citizen, such as whether one is exhibiting appropriate levels of self-esteem or has skills considered requisite for employability. Rather, I suggest that the funding models might take more account of the attachments with sustainable recovery communities that recovery-engaged arts projects might generate. Small Performance Adventures' projects demonstrate how this can be achieved both through live, in-person encounters and online via digital platforms. These attachments are formed through the lingering affects of participation in collaborative performance activities, live streams or in person events that connect people in recovery (and those curious about recovery) through public expressions of recovery communities. This offers a long-term approach to recovery, instead of transient short-term targets that do not effectively embed participants in new lifestyles of recovery.

Care-full Practices

Having offered Haraway's concept of kinship as 'inventive connection' (2016, 2) in my discussion earlier, it seems important to consider how connection and care are interlinked. Within with the field of applied theatre there has been a turn towards care as an ethico-political praxis. Amanda Stuart Fisher highlighted that socially engaged performance practices face the challenge of 'deficits of care in contemporary society' that instrumentalise and co-opt these arts practices for their own neoliberal agenda (2020, 4). Yet the process of performance practice, through its collaborative creative endeavour, is uniquely able to demonstrate the fundamental value of interdependency and, by extension, interactions of care (10).

Care, for Stuart Fisher (2020) and Thompson (2015, 2023), is an act of interrelation with another human or nonhuman. Drawing on the work of feminist care ethicists, they position care as an embodied encounter embedded in social practice (Stuart Fisher 2020, 7; Thompson 2023, 28). Their emphasis on interrelationality resonates with the discussion of recovery in this book as a practice of developing less harmful interactions with people, places and things. Recovery might then be positioned as the nurturing of care, not just towards the self, but also outwardly towards others. As critiqued in Chapter 2, the mantra of western self-help programmes reinforces an individualist approach to wellbeing that ignores the situated, interrelational realities of experiences of recovery from addiction. While in practices of recovery, such as the Twelve Steps programme, self-accountability and internal reflection is an important aspect of the process, ultimately accountability for actions with and towards others is key to moving beyond the behavioural patterns of active addiction.

Through its very title Small Performance Adventures' Terminal Uniqueness project, discussed earlier, reminds its participants to move beyond personal exceptionalism and the self-absorption that comes with addiction-based thinking patterns. Rather, through the sharing of messages, images and videos via the Facebook pages, members of this online community engaged in acts of care-full connection with others during a time of unprecedented difficulty. McCoy's introduction to the first watch party film commented on how the project not only celebrates 'our own quirkiness and specialness' but is also a reminder not to 'get bound up in our own weirdness ... and actually realise how much we all have in common'. Extending this feeling of connection to the nonhuman environment, a poem written for the film observed how the colour blue – the sky, the sea – envelopes and sustains us. These examples illustrate that sustaining *being-in-recovery* requires the practice of care-full encounters with our surroundings which can particularly be supported by attachments to forms of recovery community.

Thompson reminds us, however, that there are many forms of 'bad care' and that performative gestures of care are context and culturally specific (2023, 3). Within recovery communities, codependent patterns of care can be exhibited in what Pia Mellody et al. have referred to as 'negative control' (1989, 46–48) through which someone acquires power or validation through imposing prescriptive – and potentially unwanted – acts of care with expectations of acquiesce and gratitude from the recipient. Within the historic context of applied theatre, Jenny Hughes' discussion of workhouse plays in the nineteenth century demonstrates how early forms of social theatre were utilised as a mechanism to 'enforce prevailing middle-class ideals of respectability, good character and work upon the poor' (2016, 57). As Stuart Fisher suggests, attending to concepts of care in applied theatre practice can be useful as a 'mode of critique' (2020, 10) to examine the social politics and power dynamics in operation. Saviourism and paternalism are a concern in community-based practices; consequently, applied theatre literature addresses ethical praxis by urging for 'criticality' (Hughes and Nicholson 2016, 4), reflexivity, systems of embedded partnership and dialogue (Busby 2021, 65 and 108).

Nicholson's metaphor of theatre as a gift conceptualises care in applied theatre as acts of giving which might be conceived as 'empathetic efforts' that encourage relationships of 'imaginative identification with others' lives' (2014, 170). To give and receive a gift, however, is entangled with cultural and situational factors that complicate the simple notion of gifting as altruistic. Rather than offer an idealistic concept of care in recovery, I therefore suggest that the care-full practices discussed in this chapter are, in keeping with Haraway's kinship, an appreciation of our reciprocal obligations to create the conditions to 'live and die well with each other' (2016, 1). Care becomes an acknowledgement of our dependency on each other to create such conditions and consequently the right to survival, or 'livable life' (Butler 2015, 218), for the human and nonhuman constituents of our world. Being *care-full in recovery* is not an act as such, but instead is an ongoing process of reflexivity and accountability for how we interact, and how we appreciate our 'capacity to affect (and be affected by)' our surroundings (Duff 2016, 58).

Care can also operate as a form of activism. As Thompson argues, 'Who we care for, how we care for them, and what motivates that care, cannot be detached from the wider politics that struggles against discrimination and cruelty' (2023, 5). Care-full arts practice, such as Small Performance Adventures' OAD project, become a political gesture towards social justice. As discussed earlier, the recoverist activism of the OAD project creates visibility for the recovery community and for the experiences of those impacted by addiction, including people affected by the addiction of loved ones. By revealing that recovery is not only possible, and emphasising connection and mutual endeavour, the project further demonstrates an ethos of 'life-living' (Manning 2016, 3–8) that reminds us of our collective responsibility in contributing to 'atmospheres of recovery' conducive to healing (Duff 2016, 58).

Conclusion

Throughout this chapter kinship has been framed as a form of affective interaction that acknowledges the ways in which connection to recovery communities, or societies, supports and sustains the lived experience of *being-in-recovery*. Performance practice is uniquely able to facilitate such connections and nurture new ways of *being-in-relation* with others, both human and non-human. Such kinship is also a practice of care, through attending to the ways in which we affect and are affected by the social environments around us. Given the importance of connection and collaboration in recovery-engaged arts practices, it is timely that a more prominent network of these practices has emerged post-pandemic. The Coda that follows, therefore, marks the launch of the UK Addiction Recovery Arts network in 2022.

Notes

1 Small Performance Adventures conduct a lot of arts activities that relate to experiences of recovery from addiction and mental health issues; however, their aims deliberately reframe this as working with people 'affected by life' to subvert the marginalisation and stigma that can be associated with such difficulties by using pejorative labels.
2 See https://www.therecoveryvillage.com/drug-addiction/terminal-uniqueness/.
3 Brand has publicly advocated for a recovery approach to life, using his recovery insight to comment on current issues. This is performed through Twitter posts, vlogs, his show on Radio X and his book entitled *Recovery*.
4 Proposals for a poster campaign were submitted to the AA annual conference in 2018. A record of the proposals and a copy of the poster designs can be found on AA's European region website: https://alcoholics-anonymous.eu/posters/ (accessed 1 February 2019).
5 Quotations taken from the FAVOR UK website: http://www.facesandvoicesofrecoveryuk.org/about-us/#mission (accessed 1 February 2019).
6 This project was facilitated by Portraits of Recovery, in collaboration with Parkinson, Research Director of Arts for Health at Manchester Metropolitan University.
7 Chthulucene is a term used by Haraway to denote the current time on earth in which human existence is entangled with the nonhuman. She uses this term to challenge human-centred perspectives, instead referring to all life forms as earthly critters.
8 Fox's chapter in *Addiction and Performance* (2014) outlines in-depth two plays that he wrote inspired by real experiences from people he had met or worked with. For further information, the company website also has an archive of some of the plays he directed during his artistic directorship. See www.edgetc.org.

References

Alcoholics Anonymous (1997) 'The birth of AA, its growth and the start of AA in Great Britain', *About AA*. Available at: https://www.alcoholics-anonymous.org.uk/about-aa/historical-data (accessed 26 January 2019).

All Party Parliamentary Working Group for Arts, Health and Wellbeing (2017) *Creative health: The arts for health and wellbeing*. London: HMSO.

Baxter, V. and Low, K.E. (eds) (2017) *Applied theatre: Performing health and wellbeing*. London: Bloomsbury Methuen Drama.

Bradway, T. and Freeman, E. (eds) (2022) *Queer kinship: Race, sex, belonging, form*. Durham, NC: Duke University Press.

Brodzinski, E. (2010) *Theatre in health and care*. Basingstoke and New York: Palgrave Macmillan. Available at: http://public.eblib.com/choice/publicfullrecord.aspx?p=652444 (accessed 15 November 2018).

Bungay, H. and Clift, S. (2010) 'Arts on prescription: A review of practice in the UK', *Perspectives in Public Health*, 130 (6), pp. 277–281. Available at: https://doi.org/10.1177/1757913910384050.

Busby, S. (2017) 'Finding a concrete utopia in the dystopia of a "sub-city"', *Research in Drama Education: The Journal of Applied Theatre and Performance*, 22 (1), pp. 92–103. Available at: https://doi.org/10.1080/13569783.2016.1263557.

Busby, S. (2021) *Applied theatre: A pedagogy of Utopia*. 1st ed. NY: Bloomsbury Academic.

Butler, J. (2015) *Notes toward a performative theory of assembly*. Cambridge, MA: Harvard University Press.

Fancourt, D. (2017) *Arts in health: Designing and researching interventions*. 1st ed. Oxford and New York: Oxford University Press.

Fox, P. (2014) 'Outside Edge: Addiction recovery theatre – a theatre of survival and revolution in hard times', in J. Reynolds and Z. Zontou (eds) *Addiction and performance*. Newcastle upon Tyne: Cambridge Scholars Publishing, pp. 358–384.

Freebody, K. and Finneran, M. (2021) *Critical themes in drama: Social, cultural and political analysis*. London: Routledge.

Haraway, D.J. (2016) *Staying with the trouble: Making kin in the Chthulucene*. Durham, NC: Duke University Press.

Hughes, J. (2017) 'Theatre and the social factory', *Research in Drama Education: The Journal of Applied Theatre and Performance*, 22 (1), pp. 1–6. Available at: https://doi.org/10.1080/13569783.2017.1285875.

Hughes, J. and Nicholson, H. (eds) (2016) *Critical perspectives on applied theatre*. Cambridge and New York: Cambridge University Press.

Kewley, S. (2019) 'Changing identities through Staging Recovery: The role of community theatre in the process of recovery', *The Arts in Psychotherapy*, 63, pp. 84–93. Available at: https://doi.org/10.1016/j.aip.2019.02.002.

Manning, E. (2016) *The minor gesture*. Durham, NC: Duke University Press.

McAvinchey, C. (ed.) (2014) *Performance and community: Commentary and case studies*. London: Bloomsbury Methuen Drama.

Mellody, P., Miller, A.W. and Miller, K. (1989) *Facing codependence: What it is, where it comes from, how it sabotages our lives*. 1st ed. San Francisco, CA: Perennial Library.

Nicholson, H. (2014) *Applied drama: The gift of theatre*. 2nd ed. Basingstoke and New York: Palgrave Macmillan.

Parkinson, C. (2015) 'The Recoverist Manifesto'. *Issuu*. Available at: https://issuu.com/artsforhealth/docs/rm_online_version (accessed 3 March 2018).

Ridout, N.P. (2013) *Passionate amateurs: Theatre, communism, and love*. Ann Arbor: University of Michigan Press.

Stuart Fisher, A. (2020) 'Introduction: Caring performance, performing care', in A. Stuart Fisher and J. Thompson (eds), *Performing Care: New Perspectives on Socially Engaged Performance*. Manchester: Manchester University Press.

Taylor, D. (2003) *The archive and the repertoire: Performing cultural memory in the Americas*. Durham, NC: Duke University Press.

Thompson, J. (2011) *Performance affects: Applied theatre and the end of effect*. Basingstoke and New York: Palgrave Macmillan.

Thompson, J. (2015) 'Towards an aesthetics of care', *Research in Drama Education: The Journal of Applied Theatre and Performance*, 20 (4), pp. 430–441. Available at: https://doi.org/10.1080/13569783.2015.1068109.

Thompson, J. (2023) *Care aesthetics: For artful care and careful art*. London and New York: Routledge.

Tracy, K. and Wallace, S. (2016) 'Benefits of peer support groups in the treatment of addiction', *Substance Abuse and Rehabilitation*, 7, pp. 143–154. Available at: https://doi.org/10.2147/SAR.S81535.

6 Coda
Addiction Recovery Arts Network

On 8 September 2022, I hosted a live performance showcase within the London College of Music at the University of West London. Nine UK-based organisations specialising in arts practices with, by and for people affected by addiction convened to share a programme of performances, presentations and workshops to invited guests. The audience entailed an array of representatives from funding bodies, arts for health commissioners, addiction support professionals and members of the All Party Parliamentary Group (APPG) for Twelve Steps.[1] Also among the audience were the performers and members of the addiction-recovery arts organisations who would be showcasing their practice and were the founding members of a newly formed network. Seated around clusters of cabaret tables, with writing materials and scattered information leaflets about upcoming projects, the audience were invited to engage in conversation and take advantage of the informal networking opportunities that would emerge throughout the day. A relaxed performance style, including access to a quiet space as well as freedom to move around, was established from the start.

As Thompson observed in his discussion of the *affect* of applied theatre projects, the 'accidental' or 'peripheral' social moments can be just as impactful as the formal agenda (2011, 116). Embracing my awareness of the importance of incidental encounters, I was keen to create an environment that was conducive to social interaction in between and alongside the scheduled presentations. The overall agenda for the event, after all, was to instigate connection and raise awareness. This attention to connection was not only to share knowledge of recovery arts practices with professionals who might fund or commission this form of work, but also to facilitate the opportunity for members of an Addiction Recovery Arts (ARA) network to meet together in person.

The live sharings of performance were a powerful conduit for instigating reflection and discussion. Beginning with a premier performance of a new collaboration with New Note Orchestra and Fallen Angels Dance Theatre, the combination of live music and dance exploring themes of recovery generated a resonance that permeated throughout the day. Comments posted on the feedback wall referenced felt sensations in response to this performance, denoted by words such as raw, breath-taking, beautiful, intense. It is, nonetheless,

DOI: 10.4324/9781003271062-7

reductive to attempt to capture the experience of the performance in writing. These words, however, indicate affective interaction in keeping with the discussions throughout this book. In a documentary interview captured later in the day, I commented on the experiential focus of the programme in that I hoped people would be able to 'see and feel' what the practices were about. It would seem that this had indeed been achieved and was made possible by the generosity of those who participated in the event, enabling the staging of an atmosphere of recovery.

Performance events are particularly effective in generating what Duff has coined as 'atmospheres of recovery' (2016, 116). My first experimentation with curating collaborative recovery arts events emerged from the culmination of my doctoral research whereby I invited the artists and organisations featured in my thesis to take part in a pop-up recovery arts café-cabaret as part of the Collisions Festival at the Royal Central School of Speech and Drama in October 2019. This early prototype event examined how the cultivation of a recovery community can be instigated by shared cultural activity that directly engages with what it means to be in recovery from addiction. I also intended to experiment with the political potential of pop-up gatherings of recovery-engaged performances as a form of activism to highlight the valuable insights of those who have struggled with addiction. This was, however, a small gathering contingent upon the goodwill of the artists who had contributed to my research and was a way in which I could both celebrate their work and introduce many of them to each other for the first time. It became clear that facilitating connection and collaboration was vital in assisting the survival and growth of this not well-known, yet distinct, field of practice. The ARA network launch in 2022 was, therefore, an important extension of my earlier experimentation with collaborative recovery arts events.

The above events, however, were inevitably confined to the space-time of their location. During the discussion held at the conclusion of the ARA event, many of the audience members expressed their desire for a more formalised network presence. Initially, after the event, it was unclear as to how the network might operate and the creation of a formal structure or body seemed both onerous and not in keeping with the spirit of a recovery-engaged, fluid and inclusive cultural movement. Who should be responsible for the management of it? What would determine membership? How could such an organisation have a more explicit and, potentially global, presence? These were questions that, in the weeks following the event, seemed devoid of answers.

An unexpected answer arose, however, in the form of a proposal from Alex Mazonowicz who had attended the event as a performer with New Note orchestra. Drawing on his experience as an editing professional, Mazonowicz suggested that a publication focused specifically on recovery arts might be a good way to continue to raise awareness about these practices. A few months later, and with the support of a further grant from the University of West London's knowledge exchange seed fund, editorial management by Mazonowicz and the creation of an editorial board led by me, the first edition of

Performing Recovery was released. This digital magazine contains articles by and about artists-in-recovery or organisations working in the field of addiction recovery arts. So far, the contributions have shared insights on recovery-friendly culture and reflections on issues relevant to this area of practice and the communities represented through it. At the time of writing, the magazine had been viewed in diverse countries around the globe, including Europe, the USA, Australia and China. The directory of organisations listed within the publication had been extended to include an international page revealing new connections with practices happening beyond the UK.

Continuing Messy Connections

Throughout this book, I have suggested that the facilitation of recovery-engaged arts activity should be attuned to the ways in which the social and structural aspects of the wider society can inhibit capacities for recovery. To examine how performance-making can be imbricated with practices and experiences of recovery, I began with a discussion in Chapter 1 of what it means to be in recovery. I highlighted the experience of recovery as a personal effort towards (a never quite achieved) balance in adopting less harmful forms of feeling, thinking and doing, despite encountering moments of pain or antagonism. Recovery, in this book, has therefore been viewed as an ongoing process of personal regeneration that is best supported through connection with supportive others such as forms of recovery communities or peer networks. Consequently, recovery is simultaneously a personal and collective experience.

Manning's philosophical concept of life-living (2016, 8) has been useful to my theorising of a recovery-engaged approach to performance practice. Building on her proposition that we value life as interconnected and interdependent with others, including the nonhuman features of our surroundings, we might appreciate how addiction is a systemic issue, not simply a personalised pathology. We, as a society, should therefore take account of our collective responsibility to enable 'atmospheres of recovery' (Duff 2016, 58). I am, nonetheless, all too aware of the limited scope of any arts activity in generating personal, let alone societal, change. Yet I believe that cultural movements, such as the growing ARA network, can foster connection to and with environments that reveal and nurture crucial habitations of recovery communities amid ailing, addiction-soaked societies. Through further encounters (*messy connections*) with these distinct practices this emergent movement of recovery-engaged artistic practice will continue to unfold and reach those who might benefit from cultural environments that enhance rather than hinder recovery.

Note

1 An APPG is an informal cross-party group organised by members of the UK parliament. It does not have an official capacity, but is used to raise awareness of a

particular issue and can oversee consultations and publish recommendations regarding it. The APPG for Twelve Steps was formed to highlight evidence of the impact of Twelve Steps recovery and improve access to it. See https://www.12stepsappg.com/.

References

Duff, C. (2016) 'Atmospheres of recovery: Assemblages of health', *Environment and Planning A*, 48 (1), pp. 58–74. Available at: https://doi.org/10.1177/0308518X15603222.

Manning, E. (2016) *The minor gesture*. Durham, NC: Duke University Press.

Thompson, J. (2011) *Performance affects: Applied theatre and the end of effect*. Basingstoke and New York: Palgrave Macmillan.

Index

Abraham, Nicolas 10
accountability 52
addiction 1; 'ambivalence' to 49; assemblage of 3–5, 8; atmospheres of recovery 97; -based activity 22; -based behaviour 8; in contemporary society 73; coping mechanism for pain and distress 60; definition 5; heroin 73–74; identity 49, 52–53; -orientated behaviour 42–43, 52; psychosocial factors of 8; recovery 12–13, 24, 44, 60, 69, 77–78, 80, 86–87; research 3, 24; support staff in treatment service 67; treatment 10, 40, 56, 66–67; *see also* recovery
Addiction Recovery Arts (ARA) network 3, 113
aesthetics of care 105
aesthetics of critical visibility 54
affect aliens 81
affective attunement 40
affective economies 40, 71–72
aggressive healing 47
aggressiveness 52
agonism 53, 55
agonistic activism 52–53
'agonistic democracy' 51
Ahmed, Sara 10, 40, 65
Ahmed's concept of 'sticky affect' 61
Alchemy theatre festival 80
alcohol/alcoholism 1; consumption 2; -free social space 11; *see also* addiction
Alcoholics Anonymous (AA) fellowship 99
Alexander, F. K. 47
All Party Parliamentary Group (APPG) 99–100, 106, 113
alternative public spaces 77
Anderson, Michael 25

anger 52
antagonism 40, 50–51
anthropomorphism 64
Antidote, The 23, 26, 33–34, 39–41, 50
anxiety 2, 26–27
applied performance-making 29
Archive and the Repertoire, The (2003) 101–102
artistic practice: 'addict identity,' affective economies of 71–74; objects as narratives of repair 68–71; objects of addiction as dramaturgical tools 61–67; performance as agonistic activism 71
artists in-recovery 98
arts activity 2
arts-based activity 1, 13
atmospheres of recovery 8–14, 110, 114–115
attunement 40–41

Barad, K. 60
Baxter, Veronica 106–107
behavioural and thinking processes 9
being-in-recovery 14
Bennett, J. 60
Berlant, Lauren 31, 55
Bernstein, Robin 63
Beswick, Kate 82
Beyond Illness: Madness, Art and Society 56–57, 59
Biology of Desire, The (2016) 64
#BlackLivesMatter 2, 105
Blenheim Community Drug Project's Shine café in Haringey 11
Body in Pain, The 70–71
Brand, Russell 13, 99–100
Breaks and Joins participatory arts project 69–70
British Medical Journal 70

118 *Index*

Brodzinski, Emma 107
Brown, Brené 44
Buddhist spiritual practice 54–55
'Build Back Better' 2
Burke, Tarana 83–84
Busby, Selina 31
Butler, Judith 9

Campbell, Nancy 6, 86
Canadian Family Physician 70
capitalism 54
care: form of activism 109–110; -full in recovery 109; -full practices 108–110; *see also* recovery
Chaudhuri, Una 89
check-in and check-out contributions 29–30
chocolate cheesecake 64
chrononormativity concept 29
CIA-sponsored narcotic trade 78
civil rights issue 102–103
Cocaine Anonymous 6
'co-constellation' 21
Coda 113–115
codependency 43–44
co-habitation concept 105
collaborative arts activity 43–44
collaborative creative process 39
collaborative theatre-making process 40, 50–51
collaborators' anxiety 51–52
Colour of Injustice, The 7
community: -based practices 109; -based treatment facilities 66; drama projects 77; membership 100
compassionate mobilities 55
conflictual affective economy 86
conflictual consensus 51, 53
connection, mode of 13
consciousness 4; memory 10
constellations, concept of 44
controlling behaviour 52
COVID-19 pandemic 69–70, 91–92, 97, 101, 103
Cox, Molly 93
criminal justice 40
critical vulnerability 32
cruel optimism 55
cultural movements 115
Cultural Politics of Emotion, The (2014) 40, 73
cultural practices and values 10

decriminalisation 7
deep engagement 29
Deleuzian concept of masochism 56
Dennis, Fay 3–5, 8
digital conferencing 99
disagreement 53
disease and criminalisation 5–8
disrupting stereotypes of place and 'dangerous other' 81–87
Dolan, Jill 31
domesticity 82
dramatization of stigma 62
drug: abuse 1; and alcohol-related harm 102; assemblage 64; commodities 64; consumer 4; paraphernalia 63–64, 67; policies 73; trade 7
Drugged Pleasures 3–4
Duff, Cameron 2, 10–11, 13
dynamic and reflexive interactions 32–34

Eckersall, Peter 70
'ecology of processes' 21
Edit Sweet 98
Edwards, Ed 77
Elsevier COVID-19 Public Health Emergency Collection (2020) 2
embracing potentiality 23
emergent marginalised community 99
emotion 10, 65
empathy 84
environmentalism 60–61
epigenetic inheritance 24
ethical and political commitment 25
ethical commitments 24
ethical-political ethos 23
ethico-political decision 34
ethico-political engagement 35
ethics of out-of-jointness 35
ethnic minority backgrounds 7
Ettorre, Elizabeth 6, 86
experience of recovery 27

Faces and Voices of Recovery (FAVOR) UK 11, 99–100
facilitating dynamic 23
faculty of memory 63
Fallen Angels Dance Theatre 26, 62, 113–114
familiarity 79
'family disease' 89
Fancourt, Daisy 106
Farrier, Stephen 29
Farrugia, Adrian 3–4, 8
fear 2; and shame 52

Featherstone, Vicky 83
feeling: of anxiety 51–52; of sound, tuning in 47–50
Finneran, Michael 77
Fisher, Stuart 108–109
Fisher, Tony 53–54
Fox, Phil 15, 104
Frank, Adam 44
Freebody, Kelly 77
frustration 47

Gallagher, Michael 48
gender: behaviour 79; -specific recovery 86; violence 82
Gendering Addiction 6, 86
Global Commission on Drug Policy 7
glocalisation 78
'graft-score-use' process 9
Grehan, Helena 70
group check-in routines 51

habitation 79
habitual attunement 63
Hale, Sonya 78, 80, 85
Hall, Stuart 6, 9
Haraway, Donna 103–104
Hari, Johann 12
Harpin, Anna 59
health and wellness concepts 4
hegemonic values 40; systems of society 46–47
heroin addiction 73–74, 104
Ho, Rachel 70
Hughes, Jenny 109
human: -centred society 56; intentionality 48–49; psychobiology 22; -to-human relations 32
Hunter, Mary Ann 51

ideas of place 78–79
identity shift 9–10
immanence concept 4
immigration 53
indeterminacy 26
Indigenous Canadians in Ontario 10
individual wellbeing 2
individuation 22, 25
industrialisation 47
inequities 85
Institute of Alcohol Studies (2022) 2
instrumentalisation 24
intelligence service collusion 78
internal reflection 108

International Overdose Awareness Day 102
inter-personal exploration 29
interrelationality 108
In the Realm of Hungry Ghosts: Close Encounters with Addiction (2013) 13
inventive connection 108

Kar, Sujita Kumar 2
Kemske, Bonnie 69
Kershaw, Baz 2

Leshner, Alan 5
Lewis, Marc 1, 64
LGBTQ+ community 6, 11, 68, 100
Like Butterflies 78–85
liminality, concept of 28
liminal milieu 29–30
linguistic vernacular 79
localised pluralist democracy 71
lockdowns 1–2; *see also* COVID-19 pandemic
Lorey, Isabel 81
loss 2
Low, Katherine 106–107

macro-political systems of society 54
Manning, Erin 9, 101, 115
marginalisation 5, 81
Marsh, T. N. 10
masochistic effect 56
Mason, Simon 60
Maté, Gabor 1, 12–13
materiality 80
maximise productivity 29
Mayo, Sue 69–70
Mazonowicz, Alex 114–115
McAvinchey, C. 107
McCoy, Kate 97–98, 103
McKenzie, Jon 28
media and entertainment 40
meditation 55; and mindfulness 54; practices 48; *see also* recovery
'messy negotiation' 51
#MeToo movement 78, 83–85
micro-biotic movement 48–49
'milieu' 21
mindfulness 54–55; activities 48
minority ethnicities 40
'mode of critique' 109
moral failing 24

Narcotics Anonymous 6

National Institute for Drug Abuse (NIDA) 5–6
'negative control' 109
negative thoughts 42
negotiation 53
neoliberal concepts of health 4
neoliberal governmentality 84
neoliberal social impact agendas 26
New Note Orchestra in Brighton 11, 113–114
Nicholson, H. 41, 109
#NoGreyArea campaign 83
'noise DJs' 48
noise music 47
not-yetness 25

object-focused performance 47
O'Connor, Peter 25
O'Grady, A. 23, 32, 62, 66
Ong, Adelina 55
On Repair (2021) 69–70
Ornell, Felipe 2
out-of-jointness 47; ethics 33
Outside Edge Theatre Company in London 14–15, 43, 61–62, 87, 104
Overdose Awareness Day (OAD) project 102

Panksepp, J. 12–13
Parkinson, Clive 68
Parslow, Joe 29
past creative collaboration 41
paternalism 109
patterns 46; of care 109
Pedwell, Carolyn 84
peer support 52
people-in-recovery 104
Performance Affects: Applied Theatre and the End of Effect 30
performances 77; -based milieus 39; practice 3, 12, 43, 110; space invoked exploration 23–24; spectatorship 13
'performing agonism' 53–54
Performing Local Places Project 27
Performing Recovery 15, 115
personal: accountability 42–43; exceptionalism 98; recovery 10–11
Political History of Smack and Crack, The (2018) 77–78
political subjectivity 53
Portraits of Recovery's (PORe): participatory art project 60, 68; pop-up exhibition 68–69
positioning recovery arts practice 31

'postcolonial' critique 49
posthumanist performativity 47, 60
potentiality 23–27
poverty and social deprivation 77
practice of reflexivity 52
precarity of recovery 97
private addiction treatment 1
process of recovery 65
psychological wellbeing 6
Psychologies magazine 54
public wellbeing 1

Queen's Platinum Jubilee bank 68
Quiet Revolution, A 7

radical democracy 53, 71; Mouffe's concept of 51
radical wellness 47
Ratnayake, Sahanika 55
Realm of Hungry Ghosts, The 10
recoverist 103
Recoverist Manifesto 102–103
recovery 8–9, 47, 70; from addiction 44–45; addiction and practices of 71; arts 11–12; assemblages of 68; attachments to place 87–94; -attuned chitchat 90; -attuned connections 97; behaviour 67; commitments 44; communities 11–12, 52, 78, 97, 99, 114; -infused democracy 51–53; practices 42–43; services 11; society 98–101, 107; walks 11–12
Recovery 47–48
recovery connections: care-full practices 108–110; community-situated creative recovery 106–108; 'making kin' in troubled times 101–104; perpetual recovery and sustained relations of care 104–106; society 98–101; terminal uniqueness 98
recovery-engaged approaches 23, 53, 104, 115; arts 9, 13, 60; attunement 52; creative communities 71; ethico-political orientation 15; ethos 61; theatre practice 28; way of being 52
recovery-engaged arts 97, 107; practices 70–71, 93, 97, 105–106, 110; projects 105; work 100
recovery-engaged performances 6, 78–79, 100–102; activity 14; antagonism 50–51; attunement 40–41; feeling of sound, tuning in 47–50; -infused democracy 51–53; practices 6, 14, 60–61, 70, 79, 101–102; reflexive

process, tuning into 41–47; revealing the obscured 53–56; theatre practice 78
recovery-orientated assemblages 8
recovery-orientated ethics 33
recovery-orientated existence 21
recovery-orientated reflections 44–45
recovery-orientated reflexive practices 51
re-entering employment 11
reflexive process, tuning into 41–47
reflexive thinking 42–43
reflexivity 45–46, 53; patterns 45
rehousing 11
relapse prevention 45
Repair Centre project 71–72
Rising Voices choir in Bristol 11
risky/riskiness 66; aesthetics 62

'safe space' concepts 33
Sally Finn in Melbourne 102
Sardar, Ziauddin 25
saviourism 109
Scarry, Elaine 70–71
Schaef, Anne Wilson 2, 24
Schechner, Richard 28
Scottish Recovery Consortium 11, 99–100
scriptive things 67
Sedgwick, Eve Kosofsky 44
Segal, Gabriel 6
self-absorption 13, 108
self-accountability 108
self-awareness 41, 45
self-care 85
self-esteem 107–108
self-generated characterisation 51
self-help 55–56
selflessness 55
self-reflection 46
self-reflexivity 52
sense/sensory: of exclusion 47; interaction 9; pedagogy 32
sex/sexual: assault 82, 85; harassment 83–84; identity 101; violence 81, 86
shared humanity 86
Shonin, E. 54–55
short-term funding contracts 91
short-term memory 62
Shyldkrot, Yaron 49–50
Simondon, Gilbert 21–22
Small Performance Adventures' projects 101–102, 107–108
SMART recovery model 13
Snowfall 78
sobriety 9, 11

social: commodity 65; cultures 80–81; distancing 1–2, 92; inequalities 2; injustice 84; movement 68; and performative interactions 90; practice 108; prescribing 106; relations construct 79; and structural phenomena 4
social media: movement 83–84; obsession 1
Social Prescribing at a Glance (2016) 106
societal attitudes 56
socio-economic policy 53
solo performance 79
sonic affect 48
sonic atmosphere 50
'sonic milieu' 50
sonic performance 54
'sonic tendencies' 49
sound-emitting objects 48
sound waves 48
space: as liminal, plural and sensorial 27–32; Massey's concepts of 78–79; of potentiality 21–22
spiritual and psychological healing 55
stagnant morals 5
Staying with the Trouble 103–104
Steinberg, Matt 87
stigmatisation 81
substance misuse and offender care (SMOC) team 91
sustained connections and practices 90
systemic inequalities 86
systemic racism and social injustice 78

Taylor, Diana 101–102
Terminal Uniqueness project 98–101; Facebook page 99; initiative 104
theatre-making 23, 25
theatrical intra-activity 47
theatrical performance 10, 13
Thompson, James 30, 41, 108–109, 113
time-bound affective experience 27
Too High Too Far Too Soon 60–63, 67, 69–73
Torok, Maria 10
trade on drugs 78
transcendental meditation practices 47, 54
transgenerational haunting 10
transgenerational trauma 10
trauma 1
Twelve Steps of Alcoholics Anonymous 6

UK Addiction Recovery Arts network 110

uncomfortable and challenging behaviour 55
unemployment 77

value judgement 25
vibrant materiality 48, 69
video conferencing platforms 93–94
vital materialism 60–62, 80
vulnerability 44

Walker, Jenny 70
War on Drugs 73
Weinstein, Harvey 83

wellbeing 55
western: -centric hegemonic norms 105; culture 6–7; -privilege 24–25; recovery programmes 49; self-help programmes 108
working-class communities 77
wounds 47
Woynarski, Lisa 89

yoga 48, 54

Zontou, Z. 62

Milton Keynes UK
Ingram Content Group UK Ltd.
UKHW031421211124
451396UK00004B/42